Sports Massage

Ramela Mills and Shanon Parker-Bennett

www.heinemann.co.uk

✓ Free online support
✓ Useful weblinks
✓ 24 hour online ordering

01865 888058

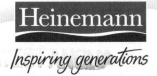

Heinemann
Inspiring generations

Heinemann Educational Publishers
Halley Court, Jordan Hill, Oxford OX2 8EJ
Part of Harcourt Education

Heinemann is the registered trademark of
Harcourt Education Limited

First published 2004

09 08 07 06 05 04
10 9 8 7 6 5 4 3 2 1

British Library Cataloguing in Publication Data is available
from the British Library on request.

ISBN 0 435 45652 0

Designed, illustrated and typeset by Hardlines Ltd, Charlbury, Oxford

Cover design by Wooden Ark Studios

Printed in Italy by Printer Trento S.r.l

Acknowledgements

Every effort has been made to contact copyright holders of material reproduced in
this book. Any omissions will be rectified in subsequent printings if notice is given to
the publishers.

Contents

Acknowledgements

Ramela Mills:

To Wes, the man who still affects my life. To my husband Kerry, my inspiration in sport, work and life. To my babies, Leilah and Owen, who always show me how proud they are of their mother. To my other son, Christopher David Mills, who through his actions reminds me that life is for living. Good friends are hard to find, but I have been fortunate to find and keep friendship and love from many who are far away, but at the same time, close. Special thanks go to those who, while I was writing this book, showed a great interest and gave support in other parts of my life: my mother in law, Jean Mills, and my friends, Jeanette Dalingwater, Ellen Adoko and Susan Pugh.

Shanon Parker-Bennett:

Many thanks to my parents Audley and Joan, and my sisters Yvonne and Natalie, for their continued support and encouragement through out my life. To my two dearest friends, Adi (Adrian) Whatling and Wendy Weddell, for always being there for Joshua and me. Thank you for your love, support, advice and words of encouragement, throughout this project and always. Thank you to my handsome young cousin Craige Coley for donating his body to 'science'. A special thanks to Patrick Skeete, co-director (with myself and Ramela Mills) of The Central Academy of Sports Therapies, for his drive and enthusiasm. Thanks to Daniel Brooks for his love and support. And most of all, a special thank you to my son Joshua, who sacrificed lots of playtime to enable mummy to complete this book. Thank you for helping mummy to press the letters on the keyboard: it took a long time, but we got there in the end!

Ramela and Shanon would both like to thank:

Leicester Stoneygate Ladies RFC for their time and patience on a very cold winter's day. Mitch Prior, Fiona Walker and Aaron Ward, who gave two days to wait for their time under the camera. All the models, including Katie Evans and Matt Fisher.

Keith at Ugo Corporate for supplying the tracksuits. A special thanks to Rabinder (Nicky) Chana and Jacquette Barnett, who gave their time to help at the photo shoot.

Pen Gresford, Julia Sandford and the team at Heinemann. Thanks also to Andy Sones – "football coach extraordinaire" – for his friendship, advice and encouragement.

The publishers would like to thank:

Trish Stableford, Karen Amos and Jeanine Connor for their valuable input.

Photo acknowledgements

The author and publishers would like to thank the following people and organisations for their permission to reproduce photographs in this book:

Neil Tingle/Action Plus 144, Glyn Kirk/Action Plus 145, Empics 148, Corbis 149. All other photographs by Trevor Clifford or Shanon Parker-Bennett.

Introduction

Sports massage is fast becoming one of the most popular areas of study within the health, fitness and sports industry. Many colleges across the United Kingdom offer sports massage either as part of a Sports Therapy Diploma or BSc Degree, a module from the National Diploma in Sports Science, or as a part-time certificated course.

Who will this book appeal to?

This book is designed to provide readers with a comprehensive, theoretical and practical reference guide to accompany any training and study within the field of sports massage. It will be particularly useful to those training to be professional sports massage therapists.

Sports coaches from any sport, whether football, rugby, gymnastics or athletics, learn how to perform pre-event, inter-event and post-event massage on the athletes in their teams. This book will also help them to gain an insight into the increased benefits that massage can bring to performance. They will also find the section on sports injuries of interest.

Qualified sports therapists and sports massage therapists will also find this book a valuable tool. They will be able to pick up new massage techniques and learn about mechanical massage instruments, as well as using it as a quick reference guide or to refresh their memory on certain aspects of previous study.

Sports massage therapist versus physiotherapist

Qualified sports massage therapists are **not** physiotherapists. A physiotherapist will have undertaken three or four years of training for a BSc in physiotherapy and might then have gone on to further study and specialization in sports injuries. Sports massage therapists are not qualified to diagnose or treat medical conditions or sports injuries. However, they are able to assist or work alongside a physiotherapist by providing specialized sports massage techniques, which may help to correct soft tissue imbalances.

Sports massage therapist versus sports therapist

A Sports Therapy Diploma is usually carried out over one or two years and a range of modules will be studied, which may include anatomy, physiology, body massage, sports nutrition, sports psychology, remedial exercise, sports injuries and rehabilitation. In addition, sports therapists may study postural analysis and corrective treatments, heat treatments, cryotherapy and the use of mechanical massagers. Sports massage plays a big part in the study of sports therapy and, as well as providing massage, a sports therapist will be taught how to recognize common sports injuries and about methods of injury management, treatment and prevention.

The benefits of sports massage

The benefits of sports massage include the following.

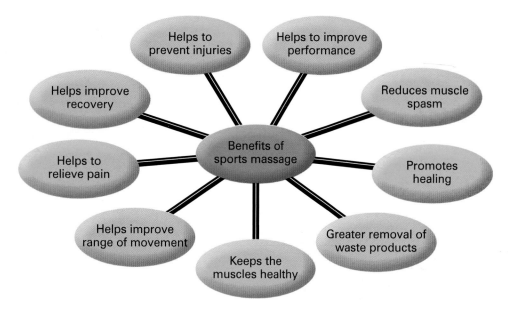

Features of the book

This book has been designed with a dual purpose:

- ☐ To provide you with the knowledge and technical skills needed for the VTCT Certificate in Sports Massage, the ITEC Diploma in Sports Massage or the Sports Massage option of the BTEC National Sports Studies qualification.
- ☐ To provide a reference book that, hopefully, you will find useful to dip into long after you have gained your qualification.

Important information about how the body works is included in the chapter called Anatomy and Physiology. Read this thoroughly before you do anything else. An awareness of the different elements that make up the human body will the reduce the chances of a massage damaging the client. The information in Anatomy and Physiology applies to many of the units throughout the book, so if you learn and understand this first, you can apply your knowledge to the practical skills you are learning.

Some helpful features

To reinforce your learning process and get you thinking, there are several features included throughout the book to help you:

Fact boxes contain a summary of important or interesting information about each section.

Massage Points explain how the background knowledge you have just read about can be related to sports massage. They show how important it is to understand the theory behind the practice.

Action Points are opportunities to apply the practical knowledge you have gained from each section.

Contraindications to Massage explain when you should be aware that a treatment might be inappropriate or needs adapting, for example if a client is injured or unwell.

Keywords is a list of the most important terms from each section. You can test yourself on defining each keyword and then check back to see how well you remembered it.

Knowledge checks are at the end of each section. These test the knowledge and understanding you should have acquired during the unit. Answering all the questions correctly is not proof that you will pass your qualification, but they are a useful form of revision.

A final word

The authors involved in the production of this book have contributed their expertise and extensive knowledge of sports massage. Their purpose in doing so is to support you in your chosen studies and to help you to develop your interest in sports massage and its application in the health, fitness and sports industry.

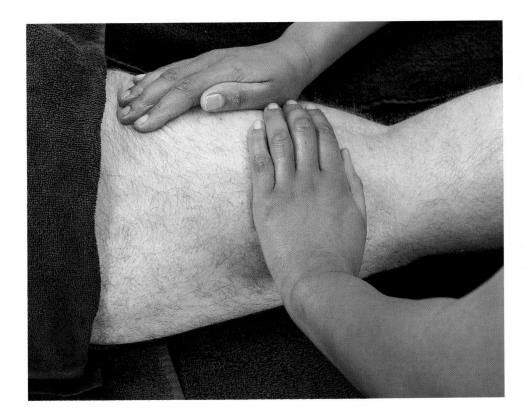

What is sports

massage?

Defining sports massage

Sports massage is an effective and beneficial form of physical therapy, not only for active sports people, or those requiring therapy after a soft tissue injury, but also for those people seeking relief from muscle tension or requiring massage for the maintenance of healthy muscles. Sports massage involves the skill of manipulating the soft tissues of the body and isolating individual muscle groups using specific and specialized techniques including stroking, kneading and compressing. The principal aims of sports massage are:

- the enhancement of a sports person's performance
- the prevention of injury
- the recovery of an athlete after an event.

Anyone taking part in regular physical activity, be it at a professional, competitive, or amateur level or just for fun, will undoubtedly encounter soft tissue problems at some stage. This is where you, the sports massage therapist, will make a difference. Your role will be to try to prevent these problems occurring, or at least reduce the risk of recurrence, by providing a regular programme of sports massage. This may include pre-event and post-event massage, mobilization and stretching. Sports massage can, therefore enhance the physical, physiological and psychological well being of the athlete.

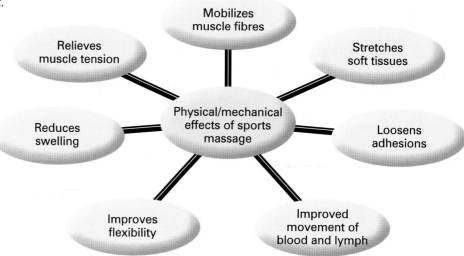

Physical/mechanical effects of sports massage

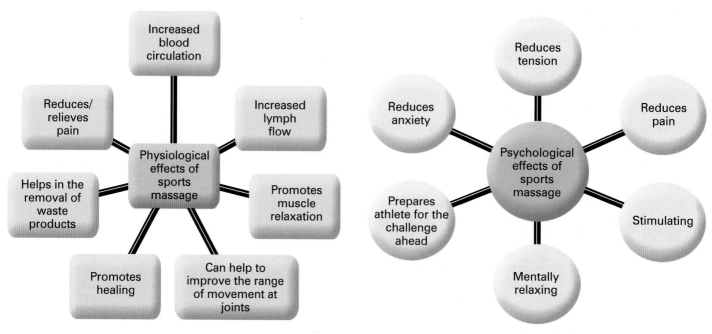

Physiological effects of sports massage

Psychological effects of sports massage

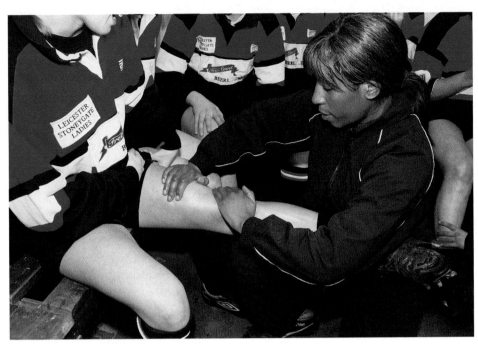

Massaging the quadriceps in a crowded changing room

The enhancement of a sports person's performance

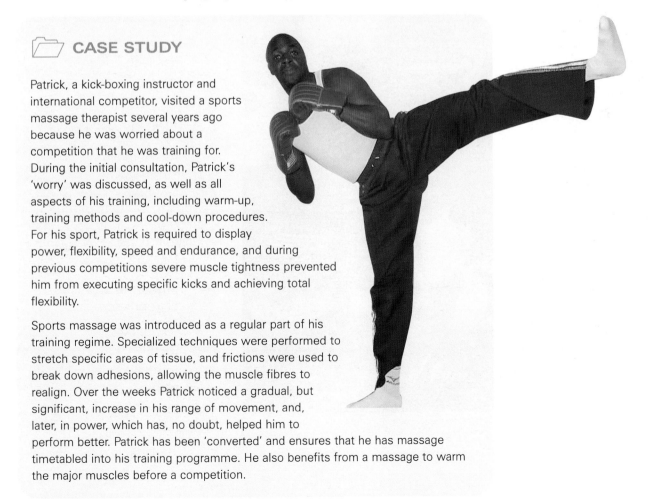

📁 CASE STUDY

Patrick, a kick-boxing instructor and international competitor, visited a sports massage therapist several years ago because he was worried about a competition that he was training for. During the initial consultation, Patrick's 'worry' was discussed, as well as all aspects of his training, including warm-up, training methods and cool-down procedures. For his sport, Patrick is required to display power, flexibility, speed and endurance, and during previous competitions severe muscle tightness prevented him from executing specific kicks and achieving total flexibility.

Sports massage was introduced as a regular part of his training regime. Specialized techniques were performed to stretch specific areas of tissue, and frictions were used to break down adhesions, allowing the muscle fibres to realign. Over the weeks Patrick noticed a gradual, but significant, increase in his range of movement, and, later, in power, which has, no doubt, helped him to perform better. Patrick has been 'converted' and ensures that he has massage timetabled into his training programme. He also benefits from a massage to warm the major muscles before a competition.

The prevention of injury

By incorporating regular massage treatments into a training regime, the therapist can help the athlete to try to prevent injuries from occurring. Massage will help the therapist to assess the condition of the muscle tissues and to provide treatment accordingly. Many athletes train daily, sometimes for between two and four hours a day, and this daily 'pounding' of the muscles could result in injury, especially if the athlete is not warming up and cooling down effectively. The athlete must also have sufficient rest periods to allow the body to recover from the stress that has been placed on it. If adequate rest periods are not taken, this will have an adverse effect on the muscles, the athlete and his or her performance. Massage alone, however, will not enable the athlete to prevent injuries from occurring.

The recovery of an athlete after an event

After an event or hard training, the muscles will probably become fatigued, due to an accumulation of lactic acid, which causes cramping and pain. At this stage, a post-event massage will help to:

- increase the flow of blood to the area
- improve blood and lymphatic circulation
- disperse lactic acid.

Sports massage therapists, depending on the level of their training, may be qualified to treat minor soft tissue injuries and aid in the rehabilitation process.

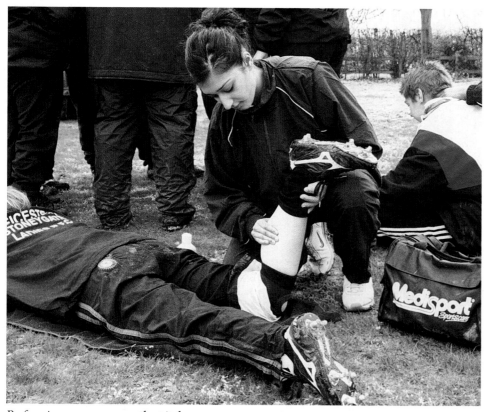

Performing a massage on the pitch

> **! MASSAGE FACT**
>
> Remember that the sports person, coach and massage practitioner will all have to work together to reduce the risk of injuries occurring or recurring, to enhance performance, and to aid recovery through:
>
> - education
> - a suitable training regime
> - correct training procedures including warm up (pulse raising, mobilization and stretching)
> - skill development
> - main activity, effective stretching and cool down
> - evaluation of performance and session
> - pre-event and post-event massage.

> **! MASSAGE FACT**
>
> Sports therapists and sports massage practitioners can be found working in many different areas of the industry including:
>
> - private practice
> - physiotherapist/ chiropractor clinic
> - health clubs
> - gymnasiums
> - football/rugby, athletic clubs
> - health spa.

Anatomy and physiology

Working as a sports massage therapist requires you to be familiar with the anatomy of the human body (its structures) and its physiology (how these structures work). As a sports massage therapist, it is very important to be able to identify body parts and demonstrate an understanding of how they work.

Exploring body systems

Before looking at the different body systems, you will first need to understand and be able to describe the movements and positions of the body.

Movements of the body

The body moves in a variety of ways that are categorized in anatomical terms: these describe the movement that the body goes through. The positions of the body are sometimes described in relation to the mid-line of the body.

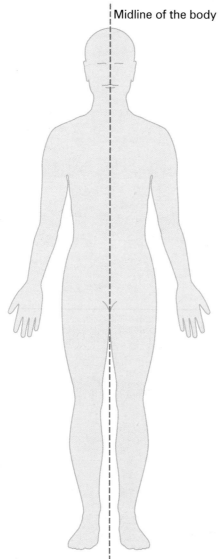

Midline of the body

Figure 2.1 *The anatomical position*

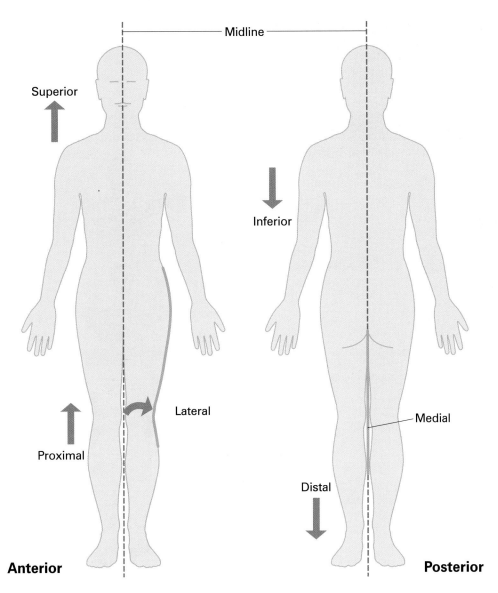

Figure 2.2 *Body positions*

Positions for sports massage

During sports massage, you may ask your client to lie in a specific position or place part of his or her body in a specific position. The position will depend on the treatment to be used. These positions are either:

- ☐ **supine** – where the position of the body or part of the body is horizontal or lying down, face up; or
- ☐ **prone** – where the position of the body or part of the body is horizontal or lying down, face down.

Your client may also lie on his or her side for some treatments.

Figure 2.3 *Supine and prone positions*

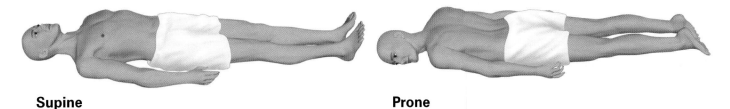

Supine   **Prone**

Describing the movements of the body

The skeletal system and the muscular system link together to create movement. The terms that are used to describe the movements that the different parts of the body perform are listed in the table below.

Movement term	Description of movement	
Abduction	Movement of a limb away from the mid-line of the body	
Adduction	Movement of a limb closer to the mid-line of the body	
Circumduction	Movement of a limb in a circular motion around the joint, giving a cone-shape movement	
Rotation	Movement of a limb towards the mid-line, thereby changing the position of the body, e.g. medial rotation, resulting in the anterior surface of the body moving medially	
Dorsiflexion	Movement of the foot towards the head, toes pointing upwards	
Plantarflexion	Movement of the foot away from the head, toes pointing downwards	
Elevation	Movement of the shoulder girdle upwards, shoulder joint to ears	

Movement term	Description of movement	
Depression	Movement of the shoulder girdle downwards	
Extension	Increasing of the joint angle of two or more bones, or where the limb straightens	
Flexion	Decreasing of the joint angle of two or more bones, resulting in a bending position occurring	
Inversion	Movement of the plantar surface of the foot towards the mid-line of the body	
Eversion	Movement of the plantar surface of the foot away from the mid-line of the body	
Protraction	Movement of the shoulder girdle forward	
Retraction	Movement of the shoulder girdle, pulling the scapulae closer together	
Supination	Movement of the forearm, resulting in the palm of the hand facing upward	
Pronation	Movement of the forearm, resulting in the palm of the hand facing downward	

▶ **ACTION POINT**

From the list of movement terms in the table, select five common movements in sports of your choice, for example, knee extension when kicking a football.

▶ **KNOWLEDGE CHECK**

1 What is the term used for body parts found at the front of the body?

2 Where would you find a distal body part?

3 What action does a body part perform when it moves away from the mid-line of the body?

4 What position would you be in if you were in a supine position?

5 What is the term for the foot turning in towards the mid-line of the body?

6 What position would the hand and forearm be in after the delivery of a dart?

7 What position would the foot need to be in to lift the body from the floor?

8 What is the body action when the head moves from side to side?

9 What shape would the hand draw if you fully circumduct the arm?

10 Name two features superior to the navel (belly button).

The skeletal system

The skeletal system provides the framework for the body. It consists of bones and the cartilage, ligaments and tendons that hold them together.

What you will learn about

☐ The skeleton
☐ Functions of the skeleton
☐ The bones of the skeleton
☐ Types of bone
☐ Bone formation
☐ Bone structure

The skeleton

The skeleton can be divided into two parts. The **axial skeleton** consists of the cranium, vertebral column and the thoracic cage. The **appendicular skeleton** consists of the shoulder and pelvic girdle, to which the arms and legs are attached (appended).

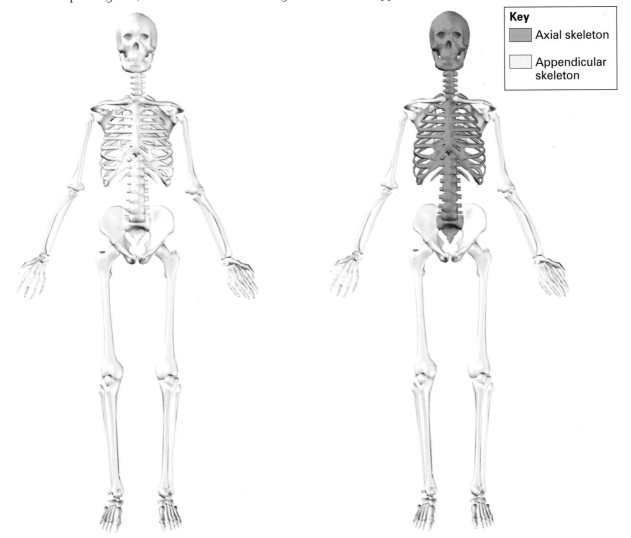

Key
☐ Axial skeleton
☐ Appendicular skeleton

Figure 2.4 *The skeleton*

Figure 2.5 *The axial and appendicular skeleton*

Functions of the skeleton

The design of the skeleton allows many different functions which enable us to live and survive. These functions include:

- **shape** – without the framework of the skeleton to provide the human body with its shape the body would be a jelly-like blob.
- **movement** – the body moves by means of the muscles and the bones working together. The muscles are attached to the bones of the skeleton to enable the lever and joints system to create movement of the body. However, other systems of the body are also required for the production of movement.
- **support** – the skeleton is required to support the visceral organs within the body. Within the network of tissues, these important organs remain in their location within the body structure. As with all of the body systems, these tissues do not work in isolation; they are attached to the matrix of the bone structure and give support to the body's organs.
- **protection** – the organs that are supported by the tissues and the skeleton also need to be protected. The organization of the skeleton's bones allows for this. Many of the internal organs are protected not only by adipose (fatty) tissue but also by the hard structure of bone. The flat bones of the skeleton provide this protection. For example, the pelvic girdle provides protection for the female reproductive organs. The cranium provides protection for the brain, especially when all of the fixed joints have fused after adolesence.
- **calcium storage** – bone is the body's largest storage tank for the mineral calcium. Calcium is stored in bone to be used for bone formation and maintenance. Calcium is also used for muscular contraction.
- **blood cell production** – the bone is structured to allow for the production of blood cells. This occurs in the marrow of the bone, which is found in the epiphysis region and the shaft (diaphysis) of all long bones (See Figure 2.6 on page 22).

The bones of the skeleton

The adult body is made up of approximately 206 bones, although at birth a baby possesses over 300. These numbers change because some of the bones that a baby has join together to form bigger single bones during their development. An example of this is in the skull where there are originally eight separated pieces of bone which come together to form a single structure to protect the brain.

Bones are constantly changing in structure and this requires the intake of certain nutrients in the correct amounts. To ensure bones develop and to maintain levels of bone density and strength, it is essential that we consume the correct amount of nutrients specific to our needs and that we participate in regular physical activity.

> **! BONE FACT**
>
> Humans are born with more bones than they die with. Some of the bones that make up the skeleton, especially those that are used for protection, fuse together to form a solid structure. One example of this is the pelvis.

Types of bone

The bones that make up the axial and the appendicular skeleton can be placed into groups according to their shape and function.

Type of bone	Example found in the body	Example of function
Short bone	Carpal; metatarsal	Small or fine movements
Long bone	Femur; humerus	Large or gross movements; cell production
Irregular bone	Vertebrae	Protection; shape
Flat, or plate, bone	Pelvic girdle; cranium	Attachment of muscle; protection
Sesamoid bone	Patella	Prevention of hyper-extension of the femur

! BONE FACT

Bones are able to become harder and stronger, through absorption of the mineral calcium, and by participation in regular exercises.

Bone formation

Ossification is the process of bone formation. The shape of a skeleton before birth is a result of soft connective tissue (cartilage) starting to take on the form of the skeleton. Bone starts to develop from these tissues during the ossification stage.

Stages of ossification

Ossification is carried out in two stages: **intramembranous ossification** and **endochondral ossification**. Intramembranous ossification is the process of bone formation that occurs at the points of tough connective tissue, for example, the tissue found between the joints of the bones that make up the skull (cranium). This tissue is replaced by bone by means of the intramembranous ossification process. Endochondral ossification is the process of bone formation that occurs where the hyaline cartilage or the epiphyseal plates are found.

Bone structure

There are two main types of bone tissue that make up our skeleton: the **compact bone** and **cancellous bone**. Compact bone is found in the shaft, or diaphysis, of long bones. It is found in the external layer of bone and helps the bone to cope with the physical stresses that are experienced throughout life. Cancellous bone is also referred to as spongy bone and is found under the layer of compact bone. Red bone marrow is found in cancellous bone.

> **! BONE FACT**
>
> The skeleton develops from the ossification stage and continues into adult life until 25 years of age.

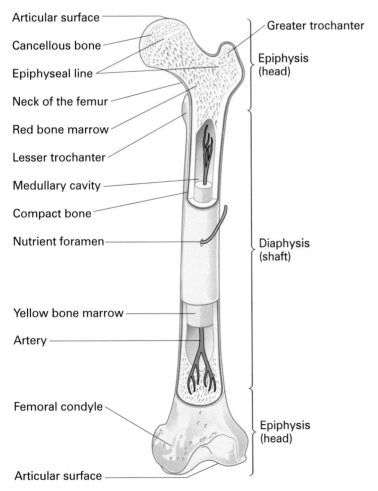

Figure 2.6 Structure of a long bone

Osteoclasts are cells that are responsible for breaking down old bone and cleaning the bone environment. This then helps the osteoblasts to carry out their role effectively.

▽

Osteoblasts are bone-forming cells. They help to develop new bone throughout life. Once they have carried out their role they become osteocytes.

▽

Osteocytes are the cells within bone that maintain bone formation. They are mature bone cells that are found within the matrix of bone.

▽

The periosteum is a tough layer found on the surface of bone to which muscles are attached. This layer is also vital for bone growth and blood supply.

Figure 2.7 *Bone formation*

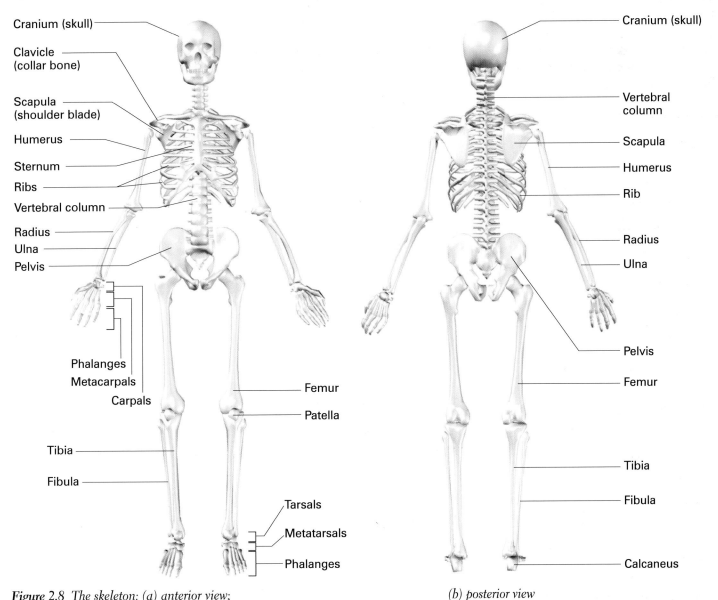

Figure 2.8 *The skeleton: (a) anterior view;*   *(b) posterior view*

The vertebral column

Posture is vitally important whether the body is static or moving. As a sports massage therapist, it is essential to acquire knowledge of the vertebral column. The vertebral column, or spine, is involved in posture, movement, stability and protection. It is made up of 33 bones that fit together to form an S-shape. Some of these bones fit together to allow for movement at these joints and some are fixed together. Between these joints are discs that act as shock absorbers.

One of the primary roles of the vertebral column is to provide protection for the spinal cord. If the cord is damaged in any way it can compromise the movements of the rest of the body or even cause death. The 33 bones that the vertebral column is made up of can be divided into five sections as shown in Figure 2.32.

The skull

The cranium, or skull, sits on top of the vertebral column, attached by a pivot joint. The cranium consists of many flat and irregular bones that give the head and face its shape.

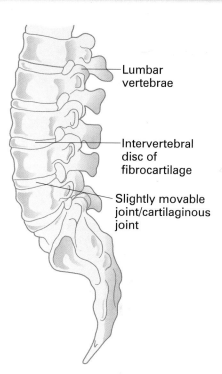

Figure 2.9 The vertebrae

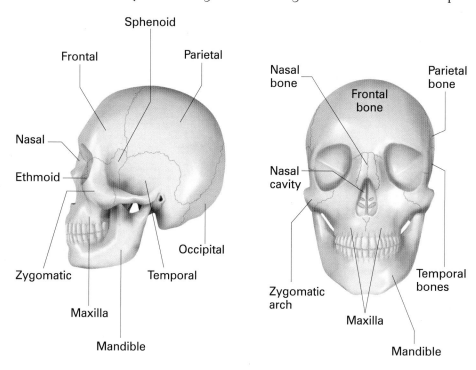

Figure 2.10 Bones of the skull

Shoulder and pelvic girdles, arms and legs

The appendicular skeleton is made up of the shoulder and pelvic girdles, the arms and the legs.

Structure	Bones
Shoulder girdle	Two clavicles, two scapulae
Arm	Humerus, radius, ulna, eight wrist or carpal bones, five hand, or metacarpal, bones, fourteen phalanges
Pelvic girdle	Three bones: the ilium, ischium and pubis
Leg	Femur, tibia, fibula, seven foot, or tarsal, bones, five smaller foot, or metatarsal, bones, fourteen phalanges

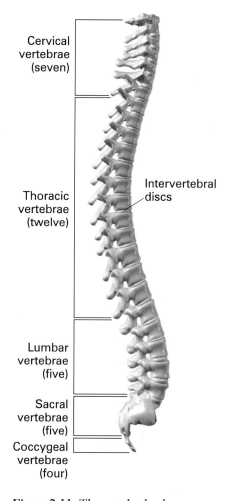

Figure 2.11 The vertebral column

Gender differences in the human skeleton

There are obvious differences in the human skeleton between genders. Females possess a wider pelvic girdle, and the flat bone that makes this bone structure is flatter in its shape compared to the male pelvic girdle. The angle of the femur from the hip to the knee joint is greater in females. This sometimes causes problems for females who want to participate in sports like long-distance running.

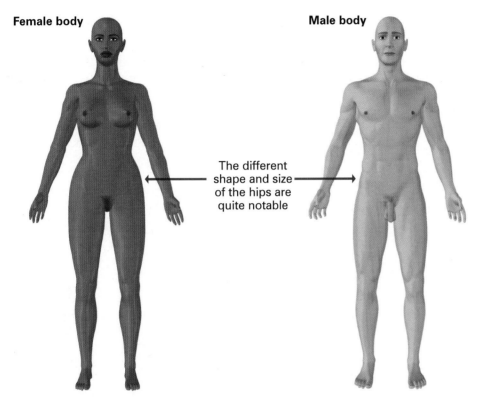

Figure 2.12 Gender differences in the human skeleton

Males are usually taller with more of a spinning-top body shape. This type of body shape tends to give males a heavier structure: there is more surface area of the body for muscles to attach themselves to, allowing for greater muscle bulk to be developed.

Joints

Joints are the points at which two or more bones meet. Bones that work together to produce movement are joined by connective soft tissues called **ligaments**. Joints need the help of muscle for the body to produce movement. The muscle pulls on the bone to make the movement happen. The muscle is attached to the bone by another connective soft tissue known as a **tendon**.

Joints can be divided into three main groups.

Type of joint	Movement	Example of joint
Fixed joint (synarthrosis)	No movement	Cranial; sacrum
Slightly moveable joints (amphiarthrosis)	Limited movement	Vertebral column
Synovial joints (diarthrosis)	Freely moveable	Ball and socket; hinge; gliding; saddle; pivot

> **! BONE FACT**
>
> Ligaments attach bone to bone. Tendons attach muscle to bone.

(a)

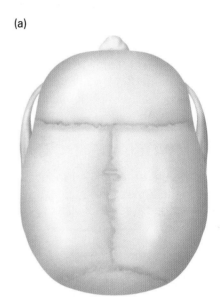

(b)

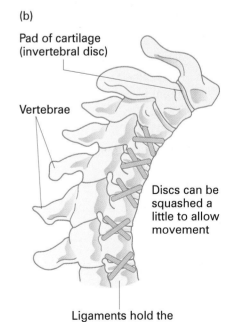

Pad of cartilage (invertebral disc)

Vertebrae

Discs can be squashed a little to allow movement

Ligaments hold the bones together

Figure 2.13 Examples of: (a) a fixed joint (in the cranium); and (b) a slightly moveable joint (in the vertebral column)

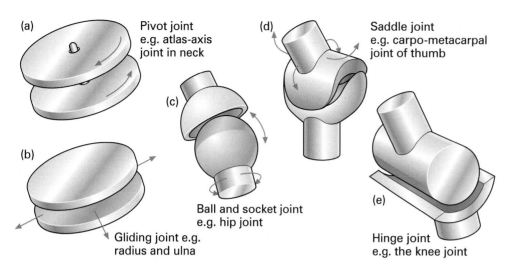

(a) Pivot joint e.g. atlas-axis joint in neck

(b) Gliding joint e.g. radius and ulna

(c) Ball and socket joint e.g. hip joint

(d) Saddle joint e.g. carpo-metacarpal joint of thumb

(e) Hinge joint e.g. the knee joint

Figure 2.14 Synovial joints

Synovial fluid is found in all synovial joints. Massage has been found to increase the release of this fluid, resulting in benefits to movement around joints, or series of joints, and the possible reduction of inflammation to an injured area or trauma spot.

MASSAGE POINT

The pressure that is produced during massage encourages blood flow to the bones. This increase of blood flow also supplies more nutrients to these areas as well as to the joints.

CONTRAINDICATIONS TO MASSAGE

- ☐ Do not apply massage over any bones that may be fractured or broken.
- ☐ Any broken or fractured bones need to be completely healed before any massage can take place.
- ☐ Do not massage any individual who may have brittle bones.
- ☐ Do not perform massage on any joint that is dislocated. Medical attention should be sought immediately for this condition.
- ☐ Do not massage over joints where there is excessive swelling and the cause is not known.
- ☐ Do not massage where there are breaks in the skin surface or fresh bruising is visible.

KEYWORDS

You should now be able to define the following keywords.

Amphiarthrosis	Diarthrosis	Osteocytes
Appendicular	Epiphysis	Periosteum
Axial	Ossification	Synovial fluid
Diaphysis	Osteoblasts	Synovial joint

▶ **ACTION POINT**

List the three types of joint. Give one example of where each of these joints can be found in the body.

▶ **KNOWLEDGE CHECK**

1 Name the six functions of the skeleton.

2 Explain the difference between a tendon and a ligament.

3 Name the two types of skeleton that make up the human skeleton.

4 Identify the five shapes of bone and give one example for each shape.

5 What is the process of bone formation called?

6 What are the growth plates of bone correctly known as?

7 Name the three categories of joints in the human skeleton.

8 Name the five different types of synovial joints in the human skeleton.

9 List the five sections of the vertebral column.

10 Which sections of the vertebral column provide movement?

The muscular system

The human body is made up of three different types of muscle tissue, each with a different function. However, the general purpose of muscles is to enable the body to move.

What you will learn about

☐ Types of muscle tissue
☐ Structure and function of muscle tissue
☐ Muscle movement
☐ Muscles of the human body
☐ Effects of exercise on muscle

Types of muscle tissue

There are three different types of muscle tissue that make up the muscular system:

1 cardiac muscle (only found in the heart)

2 involuntary muscle (also known as smooth muscle)

3 skeletal muscle (also known as voluntary or striated muscle).

Structure and function of muscle tissue

The structure and function of each type of muscle tissue are very different and each type is controlled by a different method.

Muscle type	Muscle structure	Primary function of muscle	Control mechanism of muscle	Location of muscle
Cardiac muscle	A combination of striated (striped) and smooth muscle tissue	To allow the pumping action of the heart during rest and exercise	The heart's automatic nervous system, assisted by the central nervous system (CNS)	In the heart
Involuntary muscle	Smooth	To maintain the different functions of many vital organs of the body	CNS, without conscious thought	In the blood vessels and visceral organs
Skeletal muscle	Striated (striped)	To provide movement of the body	CNS, with conscious thought	Attached to bones

Cardiac muscle is found only in the heart. The heart possesses a pacemaker (the sino-atrial node), which controls the heart rate. This rate is influenced by factors such as stress, medication, illness and exercise. These factors affect the reaction of the nervous system and influence the hormones that are released, resulting in a change in heart rate.

Involuntary or **smooth muscle** is found in the walls of internal organs (e.g. digestive system, blood vessels), and propels substances (e.g. food, blood) along. It is also called involuntary muscle because no conscious thought is required for the muscle to function.

Voluntary or **skeletal muscle** is attached to the skeleton of the human body and its major functions are to provide movement, stability and heat generation through muscular contraction. It is also called striated, or striped, muscle because of its striped appearance under a microscope. It is this type of muscle that we will concentrate on throughout this section.

Structure of skeletal muscle

As a result of a great deal of research into the structure of skeletal muscle we now know that skeletal muscle is made up of many thousands of fibres rather than just one. Each muscle in the body consists of many individual fibres, which in turn are themselves made up of even smaller fibres called myofibrils. It is within these smallest fibres that the contraction of muscle takes place. Actin and myosin are the proteins in myofibrils that are responsible for full muscular contraction.

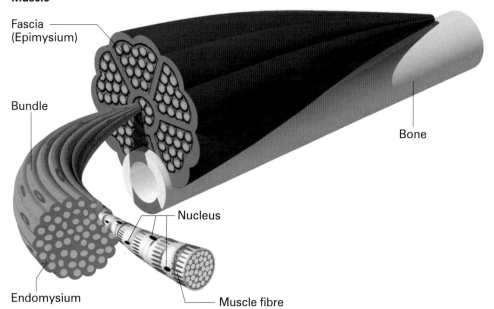

Figure 2.15 Organization of muscle fibres

> **! MUSCLE FACT**
>
> Smooth muscle tissues have more than one function for example, some aid in the secretion of hormones and in the absorption of fluids and nutrients.

All fibres are surrounded by connective tissues that give the muscle shape. These tissues also stabilize and protect the muscle. It is the outer connective tissues, known as the epimysium, that you can feel when you grasp a muscle.

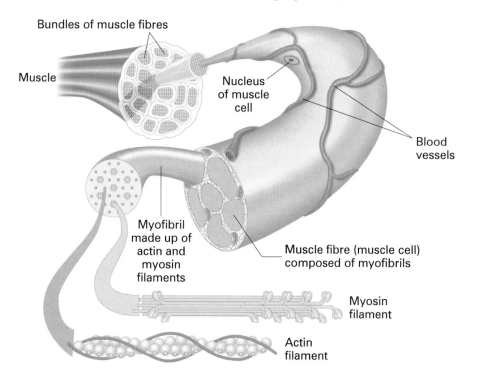

Figure 2.16 The layers of skeletal muscle

> ! **MUSCLE FACT**
>
> There are two groups of skeletal muscle: superficial muscle groups that lie just below the surface of the skin, and deep muscle groups that lie further away from the surface and beneath the superficial muscle groups.

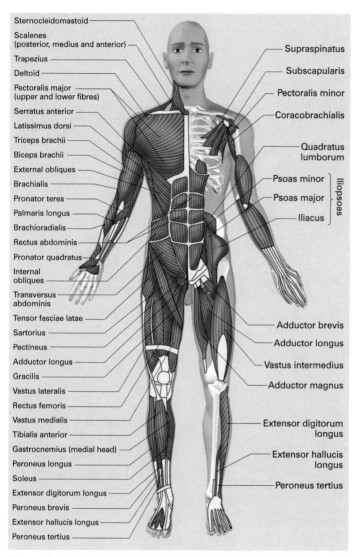

Figure 2.17 *Deep and superficial muscular system (anterior view)*

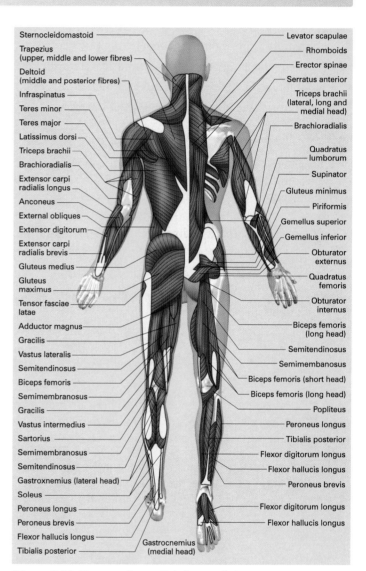

Figure 2.18 *Deep and superficial muscular system (posterior view)*

The movements of the body that we can observe are performed by skeletal muscle. The movements that we cannot observe, but can sometimes feel in our abdomen or chest, for example, are the result of other muscular tissues performing a job that we do not have to think about, that is, involuntary muscular movement.

Muscle movement

Since movement of the body is created via conscious thought processes, skeletal muscle is also called voluntary muscle.

There are many factors involved in the production of muscle movement. Nutrition is often overlooked as a factor in muscular action, but carbohydrate foods are the main fuel provider for muscle contraction. However, minerals such as calcium are also essential for the process of contraction to occur.

Characteristics of muscle tissue

Muscle tissue possesses four main characteristics:

- contractility – the ability to contract
- elasticity – the ability to return to its normal state after stretching or movement
- excitability – the ability to respond to stimuli or incoming information
- extensibility – the ability to stretch without tearing.

Muscles work in pairs; these are known as antagonistic pairs.

- Prime mover – this muscle determines the movement of an action by contracting. For example, during the bicep curl the prime mover during the flexion phase is the bicep.
- Antagonist – this muscle works together with the prime mover, but creates an opposing action. In the example of the bicep curl, during the flexion phase the triceps enables the arm to bend at the elbow joint so as to move the bar towards the shoulder girdle.

Skeletal muscle needs the use of other muscle groups called synergists and fixators for action to be successful.

- Synergists – these muscles help to stabilize the joints.
- Fixators – these muscles help to avoid unnecessary movement of the body or body part during an action.

Muscles contract to produce movement. There are three main types of muscle contraction, two where there is obvious movement and one where there is no visible movement.

1 Isometric contraction occurs when the muscle stays the same length during contraction or when the activity is being carried out. Isometric contraction occurs, for example, during the crucifix position on the rings in gymnastics (see figure 2.43).

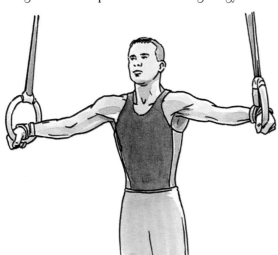

Figure 2.19 Isometric contraction on the rings

> **! MUSCLE FACT**
>
> Tendons attach muscle to bone.

> **! MUSCLE FACT**
>
> Muscles do not push; they can only pull. Muscles pull to produce movement. That is, the cells of the muscle tissue contract and then relax to their original size. The cells of the body use chemical energy to work; this energy is created from the foods that we eat.

> **! MUSCLE FACT**
>
> Muscles never really relax; they are in partial contraction and this produces the body tone.

Tension occurs in the muscle but the distance between the ends stays the same.

2 Isotonic-concentric contraction occurs when the muscle shortens when performing an action. There is obvious movement when the ends of the muscle move closer together. Isotonic-concentric contraction occurs, for example, during the upward phase of the bicep curl (see figure 2.20).

3 Isotonic-eccentric contraction occurs when the muscles lengthen under tension during obvious movement. The ends of the muscle move further away during an action. Isotonic-eccentric contraction occurs, for example, when the bicep lengthens during the downward phase of a pull-up (see figure 2.21).

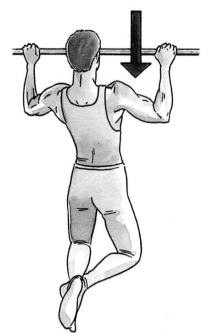

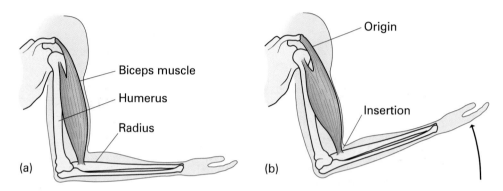

Figure 2.20 *(a) Isotonic-concentric and (b) Isotonic-eccentric contraction during the upward phase of a bicep curl*

Figure 2.21 *Isotonic-eccentric contraction during the downward phase of a pull-up*

▶ **ACTION POINT**

List the prime mover and the antagonistic muscles used in the following sports skills.

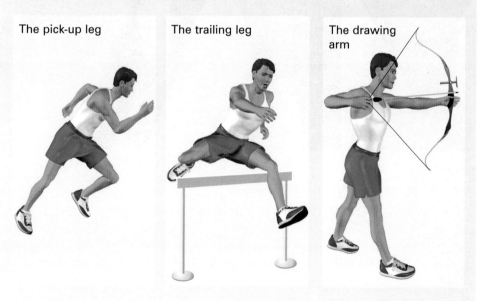

The pick-up leg

The trailing leg

The drawing arm

Figure 2.22

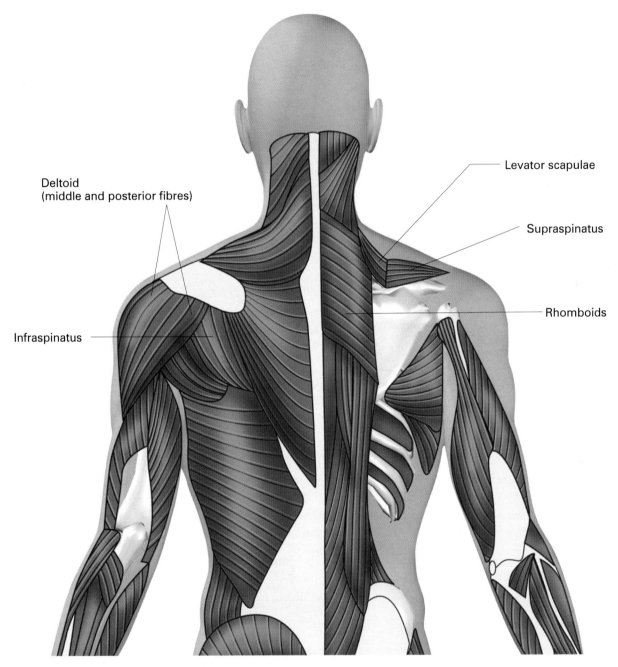

Deltoid
(middle and posterior fibres)

Infraspinatus

Levator scapulae

Supraspinatus

Rhomboids

Figure 2.23 *Muscles of the upper torso (posterior view)*

Muscles of the human body

Levator scapulae

Origin: the upper four cervical vertebrae
Insertion: upper part of the vertebral border of the scapula
Action: elevates and rotates the scapula

Rhomboideus major

Origin: from the second to the fifth thoracic vertebrae
Insertion: vertebral border of the scapula
Action: supports the shoulder and rotates the scapula

Rhomboideus minor

Origin: first thoracic vertebrae
Insertion: vertebral border of the scapula
Action: supports the shoulder and rotates the scapula

Deltoid

Origin: lateral third of clavicle, acromion and spine of scapula
Insertion: deltoid tuberosity of humerus
Action: abducts the shoulder joint, posterior fibres extend and laterally rotate shoulder, anterior fibres flex and medially rotate the shoulder

Origin is identical to the insertion of the trapezius

Supraspinatus 'rotator cuff'

Origin: supraspinatus fossa of scapula
Insertion: greater tubercle of humerus – superior facet
Action: abducts the humerus, stabilizes head of humerus in glenoid cavity;
medially rotates humerus, draws it forward and down when arm is raised;
deep to trapezius – runs underneath the acromion (only rotator cuff muscle that does not rotate)

Infraspinatus 'rotator cuff'

Origin: infraspinous fossa of scapula
Insertion: greater tubercle of humerus – middle facet
Action: laterally rotates, adducts, extends the shoulder, stabilizes head of humerus in glenoid cavity

Subscapularis 'rotator cuff'

Origin: subscapular fossa of the scapula
Insertion: lesser tubercle of the humerus
Action: medially rotates shoulder joint, stabilizes head of humerus in glenoid cavity

Most often the culprit in 'frozen shoulder'

Scalenes – anterior, medius, posterior

Origin: anterior – transverse processes of C3–C6; medius – transverse processes of C2–C7; posterior – transverse processes of C5–C7
Insertion: anterior – first rib; medius – first rib; posterior – second rib
Action: bilaterally – elevate ribs during inspiration;
unilaterally – with rib fixed, laterally flex the neck, rotate head and neck to opposite side;
anterior – flex the neck

Brachial plexus and subclavian artery pass between the medius and anterior scalene

! MUSCLE FACT

Abbreviations in these descriptions refer to different parts of the spinal column.

C = cervical vertabrae

T = thoric vertabrae

L = lumbar vertabrae.

See figure 2.11 for positions.

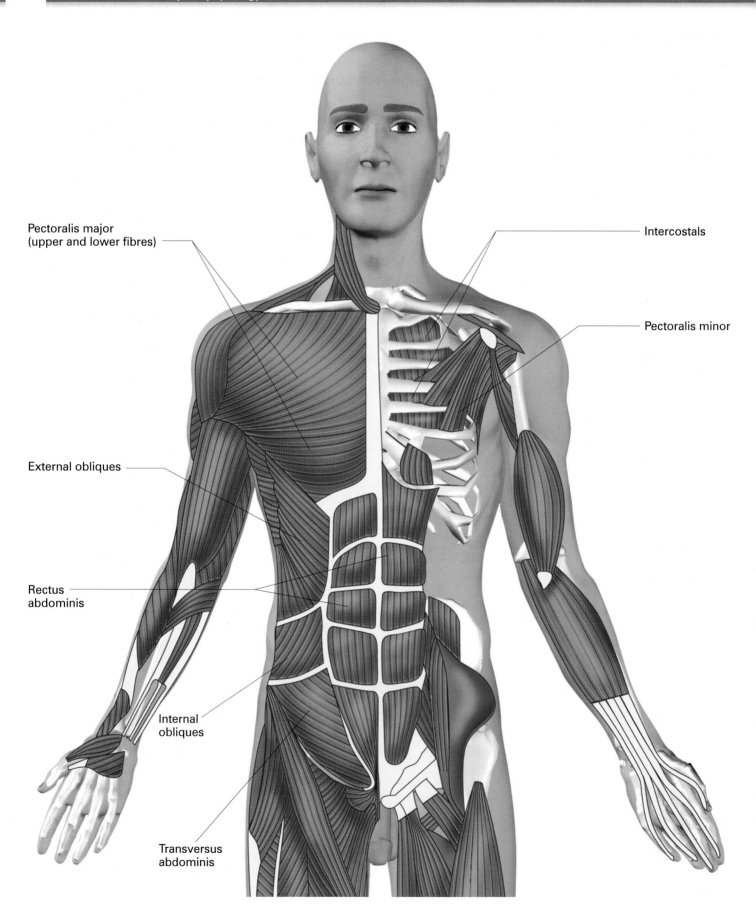

Pectoralis major
(upper and lower fibres)

Intercostals

Pectoralis minor

External obliques

Rectus
abdominis

Internal
obliques

Transversus
abdominis

Figure 2.24 Muscles of the upper torso (anterior view)

Muscles of the thoracic region

Pectoralis major

Origin: sternal half of clavicle, sternum to seventh rib, aponeurosis of external oblique muscle

Insertion: crest of greater tubercle of humerus, lateral lip of bicipital groove

Action: clavicular (upper) fibres – flexion of humerus;

sternocostal (middle and lower) fibres – extension of humerus returning from flexion;

adduction, medial rotation

Upper and lower muscle groups work in opposition, making it an antagonist muscle group to itself. For example, as the upper muscle group contracts, the lower group relaxes

Pectoralis minor

Origin: third, fourth and fifth ribs

Insertion: coracoid process of scapula

Action: slight movement of the scapula forward, depresses and abducts scapula

Pulls shoulder forward when rhomboids are weak

Intercostals

Origin: inferior and inner border of the upper eleven pairs of ribs

Insertion: superior border of the upper eleven pairs of ribs

Action: external intercostals – move the ribs upward and outwards during inspiration of air to increase the thoracic cavity space;

internal intercostals – move the ribs downward, decreasing the space of the thoracic cavity

The intercostal muscles stabilize the rib cage and assist the respiratory structures during breathing. These muscles can be described as the meat of spare ribs

Muscles of the abdominal wall

Rectus abdominis

Origin: crest of the pubis, pubic symphysis

Insertion: cartilage of the fifth, sixth and seventh ribs and ziphoid process

Action: flexes the vertebral column

Sometimes origin and insertion are reversed

External obliques

Origin: lower eight ribs (5–12)

Insertion: anterior part of iliac crest

Action: bilaterally – flex thorax and compress abdominal contents;

unilaterally – laterally flex spine and rotate spine to opposite side

Work together with serratus anterior. The direction of the fibres is the same as that of a hand being put in a trouser pocket. That is, downward and towards the mid-line of the body

Internal obliques

Origin: lateral inguinal ligament, anterior iliac crest, thoracolumbar aponeurosis

Insertion: cartilage of lower six ribs (7–12), abdominal aponeurosis to linea alba

Action: bilaterally – flex the thorax, compress abdominal contents;

unilaterally – laterally flex spine and rotate trunk to same side

Transverse abdominis

Origin: lateral inguinal ligament, anterior iliac crest, thoracolumbar fascia, cartilage of lower six ribs (7–12)

Insertion: abdominal aponeurosis to linea alba

Action: compresses abdominal contents

Deepest layer of abdominals – runs horizontally and towards the mid-line of the body

Origin: lateral supracondylar ridge of humerus

Insertion: styloid process of radius

Action: flexes forearm (handshake position)

Psoas major

Origin: lumbar vertebrae, T12–L5; bodies and transverse processes

Insertion: lesser trochanter of femur

Action: flexes hip

Provides support for the spine and maintains disc space when functioning properly

Iliacus

Origin: iliac fossa

Insertion: lesser trochanter of the femur

Action: flexes, laterally rotates and adducts the hip

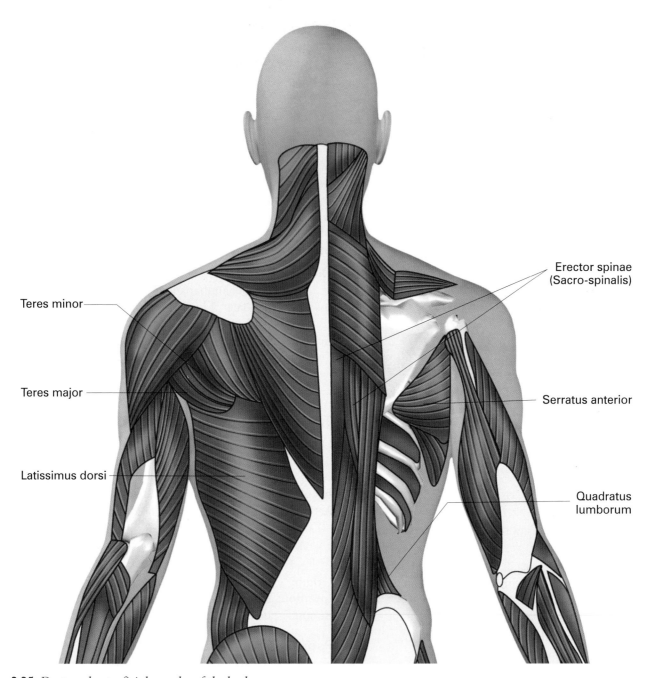

Teres minor

Teres major

Latissimus dorsi

Erector spinae
(Sacro-spinalis)

Serratus anterior

Quadratus
lumborum

Figure 2.25 *Deep and superficial muscles of the back*

Latissimus dorsi

Origin: lower six thoracic vertebrae, through the lumbar dorsal fascia from the lumbar vertebrae and iliac crest

Insertion: bicipital groove of the humerus

Action: draws the arm backward, adducts and rotates the arm inward

Sacro-spinalis (erector spinae)

Origin: sacrum and the iliac crest with additional fibres from the ribs and the lower vertebrae

Insertion: ribs, vertebrae and the mastoid process

Action: extends the trunk when both sides work together

Divides into three columns – the ilio (costo), cervicalis longissimus and spinalis

Teres minor 'rotator cuff'

Origin: superior half of lateral border of scapula

Insertion: greater tubercle of humerus, lowest facet

Action: laterally rotates, adducts, extends the shoulder, stabilizes head of humerus in glenoid cavity

Teres major

Origin: inferior angle of scapula

Insertion: medial lip of bicipital groove of humerus

Action: adducts and medially rotates humerus and draws it back

Serratus anterior

Origin: outer surface of ribs 1–8

Insertion: anterior medial border of scapula

Action: abducts and upwardly rotates scapula, holds scapula against thoracic wall

Weakness causes winged scapula. Tightness may cause 'a stitch in the side'

Quadratus lumborum

Origin: posterior iliac crest, iliolumbar ligament

Insertion: last rib, transverse processes of L1–L4

Action: bilaterally – extends the spine;

unilaterally – laterally flexes lumbar spine;

with spine fixed – elevates hip (hikes hip up);

holds twelfth rib against the pull of the diaphragm

Composed of groups of fibres: iliocostal fibres run from medial upper crest of ilium and iliolumbar ligament upward to twelfth rib (vertical); iliolumbar fibres run from the ilium to the transverse processes of L1–L4

Brachioradialis

Origin: lateral supracondylar ridge of humerus
Insertion: styloid process of radius
Action: flexes forearm (handshake position)

Triceps brachii

Origin: long head – infraglenoid tubercle of scapula
                lateral head – posterior surface of proximal
                half of humerus
Insertion: all heads – olecranon process of ulnar
Action: long head – extends and adducts the
                shoulder;
                all heads – extend the forearm from the
                elbow

Supinator

Origin: lateral epicondyle of humerus, posterior
                ulna
Insertion: proximal anterior shaft of humerus
Action: supinates forearm

Extensor digitorum

Origin: common extensor tendon from lateral
                epicondyle of humerus
Insertion: dorsal surface of middle and distal
                phalanges 2–5 (four fingers)
Action: extends four fingers, assists in extension of
                the wrist

Extensor carpi radialis longus

Origin: lateral supracondylar ridge of humerus
Insertion: base of second metacarpal bone dorsal side
Action: extends and abducts the wrist, flexes the
                elbow

Extensor carpi radialis brevis

Origin: lateral epicondyle of humerus
Insertion: dorsal surface of base of third metacarpal
                bone
Action: extends and assists in abduction of the wrist

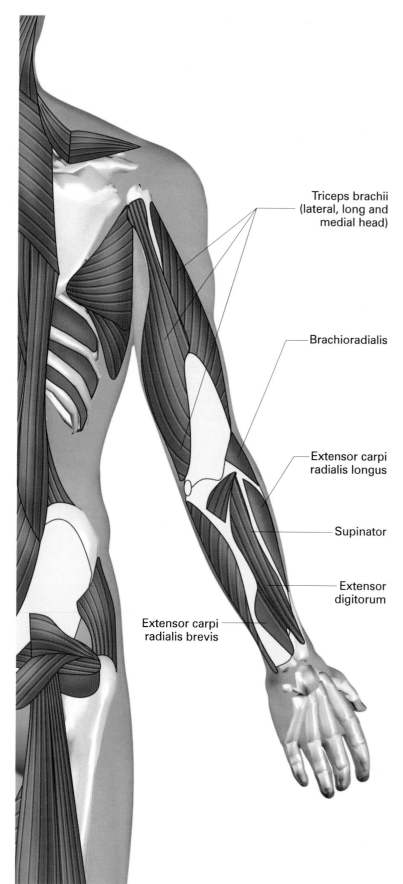

Triceps brachii
(lateral, long and
medial head)

Brachioradialis

Extensor carpi
radialis longus

Supinator

Extensor
digitorum

Extensor carpi
radialis brevis

Figure 2.26 Muscles of the arm (posterior view)

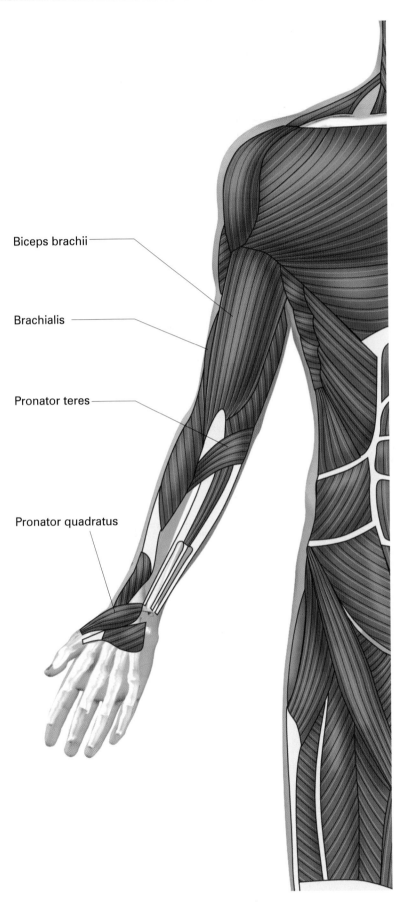

Pronator teres

Origin: medial epicondyle of humerus, coronoid process of ulna
Insertion: middle of lateral surface of radius
Action: pronates the forearm and assists in flexion of the elbow

Pronator quadratus

Origin: distal anterior aspect of the ulna
Insertion: distal aspect of the radius
Action: pronates the forearm

Biceps brachii

Origin: short head – coracoid process of scapula; long head – supraglenoid tubercle of scapula
Insertion: tuberosity of the radius and aponeurosis of biceps brachii
Action: flexes elbow, supinates forearm, flexes shoulder joint

Brachialis

Origin: distal half of the anterior surface of humerus
Insertion: tuberosity and coronoid process of ulna
Action: flexes the elbow

Biceps brachii

Brachialis

Pronator teres

Pronator quadratus

Figure 2.27 Muscles of the arm (anterior view)

Tensor fascia latae

Origin: anterior iliac crest (posterior to anterior superior iliac spine)
Insertion: iliotibial band, which continues to attach to lateral condyle of tibia
Action: flexes (internally), rotates and abducts thigh, prevents collapse of extended knee in walking

Sartorius

Origin: anterior superior iliac spine
Insertion: upper medial shaft of tibia
Action: assists with flexion, abduction, lateral rotation of hip, and with the flexion and medial rotation of knee

Rectus femoris

Origin: anterior inferior iliac spine, ilium on upper margin of acetabulum
Insertion: patella, patellar ligament to tibial tuberosity
Action: extends the knee, assists with the flexion of the hip
This is the only hip flexor of quad group

Vastus medialis

Origin: linea aspera of posterior femur
Insertion: patella, patellar ligament to tibial tuberosity
Action: extends knee

Vastus lateralis

Origin: linea aspera of posterior femur
Insertion: patella, patellar ligament to tibial tuberosity
Action: extends knee

Vastus intermedius

Origin: anterior and lateral femoral shaft
Insertion: patella, patellar ligament to tibial tuberosity
Action: extends knee

Pectineus

Origin: superior ramus of pubis
Insertion: pectineal line of femur
Action: flexes hip, adducts thigh, medially rotates the thigh

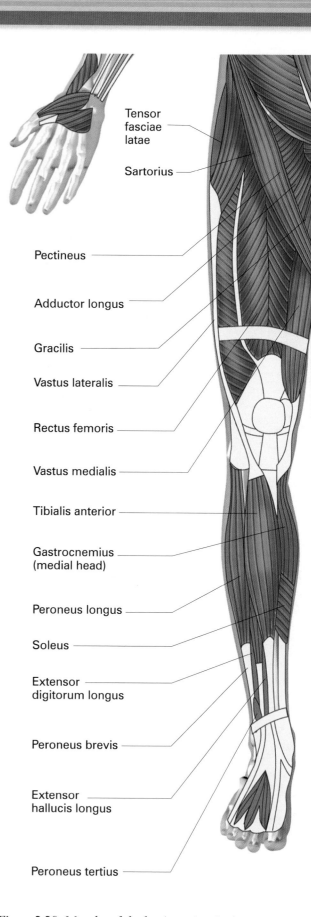

Tensor fasciae latae

Sartorius

Pectineus

Adductor longus

Gracilis

Vastus lateralis

Rectus femoris

Vastus medialis

Tibialis anterior

Gastrocnemius (medial head)

Peroneus longus

Soleus

Extensor digitorum longus

Peroneus brevis

Extensor hallucis longus

Peroneus tertius

Figure 2.28 Muscles of the leg (anterior view)

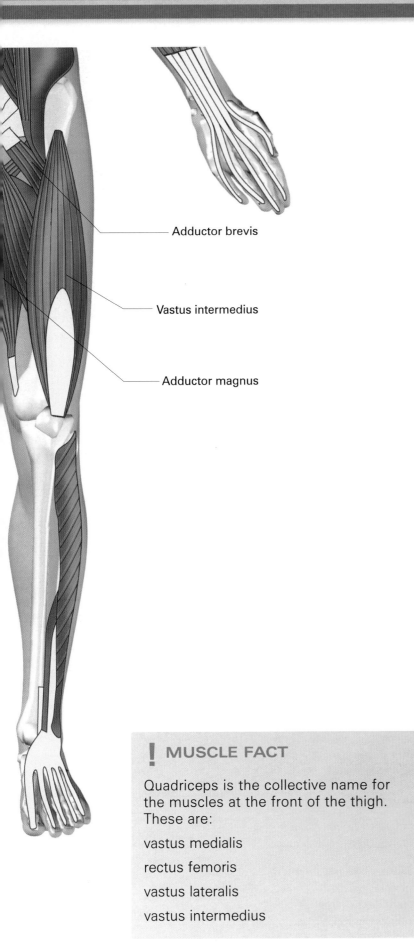

Adductor brevis

Vastus intermedius

Adductor magnus

Adductor longus

Origin:	anterior pubis just inferior to pubic tubercle
Insertion:	linea aspera of posterior femur
Action:	adducts hip, assists in flexion and medial rotation of hip

Adductor brevis

Origin:	anterior pubis
Insertion:	linea aspera of posterior femur
Action:	adducts hip, assists in flexion and medial rotation of hip

Gracilis

Origin:	anterior pubis
Insertion:	medial proximal tibia
Action:	adducts hip, assists in flexion and medial rotation of flexed knee

Adductor magnus

Origin:	inferior pubic ramus, ischial ramus, ischial tuberosity
Insertion:	proximal third of linea aspera of posterior femur, adductor tubercle
Action:	adducts hip, assists in flexion of hip, posterior fibres assists in extension of hip
	This group assists the hamstrings

Gastrocnemius

Origin:	medial epicondyle of femur, lateral epicondyle of femur
Insertion:	calcaneus via Achilles tendon
Action:	plantarflexes foot at ankle, flexes knee

Tibialis anterior

Origin:	lateral tibia, proximal lateral surface of tibia, interosseous membrane
Insertion:	medial cuneiform, first metatarsal
Action:	inverts foot, dorsiflexes ankle

Extensor digitorum longus

Origin:	lateral tibial condyle, fibula
Insertion:	dorsal surface of phalanges 2–5
Action:	extends toes 2–5, dorsiflexes the ankle, everts the foot

Extensor hallucis longus

Origin:	medial aspect of the fibula, interosseous membrane
Insertion:	distal phalanx of big toe
Action:	extends the big toe, dorsiflexes the ankle, inverts the foot

---

! MUSCLE FACT

Quadriceps is the collective name for the muscles at the front of the thigh. These are:

vastus medialis

rectus femoris

vastus lateralis

vastus intermedius

Gluteus maximus

Origin: posterior ilium, sacrum, coccyx

Insertion: femur (greater trochanter) and iliotibial band

Action: forcefully extends hip, laterally rotates extended hip, abducts hip (IT band), lower fibres (inserting on trochanter) adduct hip

This large muscle helps to stabilize the knee

Gluteus medius

Origin: ilium between posterior and anterior gluteal lines (below crest)

Insertion: greater trochanter of femur

Action: abducts and rotates thigh medially (internally), abducts, flexes and extends the hip

This section of the gluteals helps to stabilize the pelvis

Piriformis

Origin: anterior surface of the sacrum

Insertion: greater trochanter of femur

Action: externally rotates femur

Gluteus minimus

Origin: posterior ilium between anterior and inferior gluteal lines

Insertion: anterior surface of greater trochanter of femur

Action: abducts and medially (internally) rotates thigh, stabilizes pelvis on femur

Along with the gluteus medius, the gluteus minimus helps to stabilize the pelvis

Biceps femoris

Origin: long head – ischial tuberosity; short head – lateral lip of linea aspera

Insertion: head of the fibula

Action: flexes knee, extends hip, moves the pelvis slightly towards the posterior side of the body and laterally rotates the femur

Semitendinosus

Origin: ischial tuberosity

Insertion: proximal, medial condyle of the tibia

Action: flexes knee, extends hip, moves the pelvis slightly towards the posterior side of the body and medially rotates the femur

This muscle possesses a superficial, stringy, tendinous attachment

Semimembranosus

Origin: ischial tuberosity

Insertion: proximal, medial condyle of the tibia

Action: flexes knee, extends hip, moves the pelvis slightly towards the posterior side of the body and medially rotates the femur

Flexor digitorum longus

Origin: lower two-thirds of tibia

Insertion: four outer phalanges plantar surface, alongside ankle

Action: plantarflexes and inverts foot, flexes toes 2–5

Flexor hallicus longus

Origin: inferior two-thirds of posterior fibula

Insertion: plantar surface of big toe

Action: flexes big toe, weakly plantarflexes the ankle, inverts foot

Deep lateral rotators

(Superior and inferior gemelli, obturator internus and externus, quadratus femoris)

Origin: ischium, obturator foramen

Insertion: trochanter

Action: laterally rotates thigh, stabilizes the hip

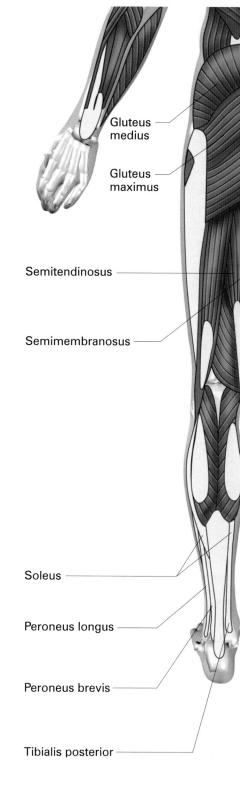

Figure 2.29 *Muscles of the leg (posterior view)*

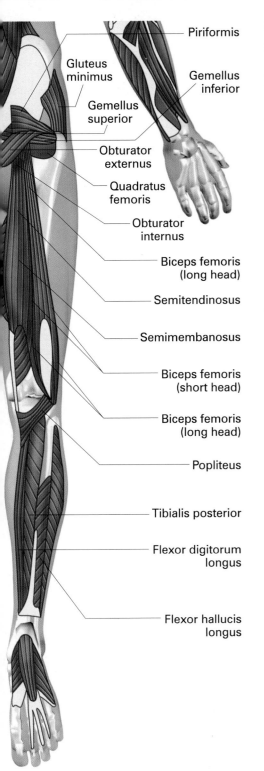

Piriformis

Gluteus
minimus

Gemellus
inferior

Gemellus
superior

Obturator
externus

Quadratus
femoris

Obturator
internus

Biceps femoris
(long head)

Semitendinosus

Semimembanosus

Biceps femoris
(short head)

Biceps femoris
(long head)

Popliteus

Tibialis posterior

Flexor digitorum
longus

Flexor hallucis
longus

Soleus

Origin: upper fibula, soleal line of tibia

Insertion: calcaneus via Achilles tendon

Action: plantarflexes foot

Deep to gastrocnemius, but wider than gastrocnemius; strong contractions pump blood from leg to heart

Plantaris

Origin: above the lateral head of gastrocnemius on femur

Insertion: calcaneus via Achilles tendon

Action: weakly plantarflexes the foot at ankle

Popliteus

Origin: lateral femoral condyle

Insertion: posterior tibial surface above soleal line

Action: laterally rotates femur, flexes the knee, unlocks knee from an extended position

Tibialis posterior

Origin: proximal posterior tibia, interosseous membrane, medial fibula

Insertion: navicular, cuneiform, cuboid bones and bases of second to fourth metatarsals

Action: inverts the foot, plantarflexes the ankle

Peroneus longus

Origin: upper lateral fibula

Insertion: medial cuneiform, plantar surface of cuboid, base of first metatarsal

Action: everts and abducts foot, weakly plantarflexes foot

Peroneus brevis

Origin: lower, lateral two-thirds of fibula

Insertion: fifth metatarsal

Action: everts and abducts the foot, weakly plantarflexes foot

---

！ MUSCLE FACT

Hamstrings is the collective name for the muscles at the back of the thigh. These are:

biceps femoris

semitendinosus

semimembranosus.

Muscles of the head and neck

Sternocleidomastoid

Origin: manubrium of sternum, medial third of clavicle
Insertion: mastoid processes of temporal bone
Action: unilaterally – lateral flex to same side and rotation to opposite side;
bilaterally – flexes head and neck

In prone position – when head is turned to side and lifted towards ceiling
– sternocleidomastoids should be prominent

Trapezius

Origin: occipital bone and all of the thoracic vertebrae
Insertion: clavicle and the spine of the scapula
Action: elevates the shoulder and rotates the scapula. It also helps to secure the
scapula

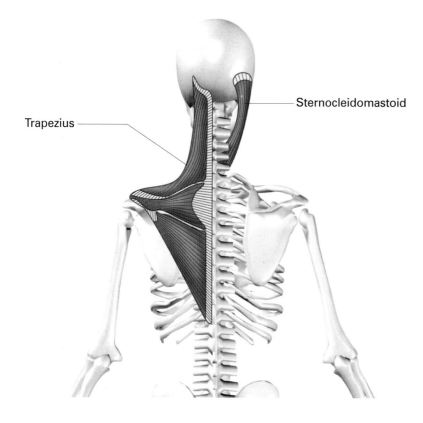

Figure 2.30 Muscles of the head and neck

Effects of exercise on muscle

During exercise there is an increase of blood flow to the working muscles. This
supplies the muscle tissue with the extra oxygen and fuel it needs for the movement
to take place. The increase in blood flow also helps to remove waste products like
carbon dioxide and lactic acid.

Any muscular or organ activity requires energy. The energy for muscular contraction
is provided by adenosine triphosphate (ATP). ATP is formed when one molecule of
adenosine joins together with three phosphate molecules. There is a very limited

supply of ATP in the body (one minute's worth at rest) but it is constantly being regenerated by the body's three energy systems:

1 ATP-PC

2 Anaerobic system

3 Aerobic system

Depending on the intensity and duration of exercise, one, two or even all three systems can work together to provide the body with energy.

The waste products lactic acid and carbon dioxide also increase during exercise and these need to be removed. If these waste products are not removed, the muscles become tired and breathing rate increases, eventually stopping the body from being able to continue with the activity.

MASSAGE POINT

Massage increases the blood supply to the muscles by three times – this helps to feed the muscles with the nutrients that they need as well as helping to remove waste products that can become harmful to the muscle tissue.

Massage helps to dispel hard knots within muscle caused by muscle spasm that may have occurred from experiencing tension and emotional and/or physical trauma. Massage can make the muscular area feel relaxed and more elastic; this may be a result of massage warming the area and manipulating the muscles that have become tense.

Through various massage techniques, some muscles that are found over joints can be stretched and loosened to increase movement where injury may have affected or limited movement of these joints.

CONTRAINDICATIONS TO MASSAGE

☐ Do not massage over a muscle believed to have been torn during the acute phase of the injury.

☐ Do not massage over a fresh bruise.

KEYWORDS

You should now be able to define the following keywords.

adenosine triphosphate	excitability	sino-atrial node
antagonistic muscle	extensibility	skeletal muscle
contractility	involuntary muscle	
elasticity	perimysium	

! MUSCLE FACT

Carbohydrates are the body's fuel for muscle action and some of the substances broken down from carbohydrates through digestive processes are stored in the muscle itself. This enables rapid muscle contraction. Carbohydrates need to be broken down to adenosine triphosphate (ATP).

▶ KNOWLEDGE CHECK

1 Name the three types of muscle tissue found in the body.

2 Give one example of each of the muscle tissues identified in Question 1.

3 Name three functions of skeletal muscle.

4 Name the three layers of skeletal muscle. Use a diagram to assist you in your answer.

5 What is the soft tissue that surrounds muscle called?

6 What is ATP and what is it used for?

7 Where would you find the anterior tibialis?

8 What is the prime mover in elbow flexion?

9 What is the antagonist in elbow extension?

The cardiovascular system

The cardiovascular system is the body's delivery system. The cardiovascular system is made up of three main parts: the heart, blood vessels and blood. Blood moves from the heart and delivers oxygen and nutrients to every part of the body. On the return trip, the blood picks up waste products for removal from the body.

What you will learn about

☐ The heart

☐ Blood vessels

☐ Blood

The heart

The heart is a muscular pump, the size of a clenched fist, that can increase in either size or thickness as a result of training. It is made up of special cardiac muscle that contracts regularly without tiring. Cardiac muscle becomes bigger and stronger if regular exercise is carried out. This means the heart is more efficient at pumping blood around the body.

> **! HEART FACT**
>
> The heart has its own neural control. If the central nervous system is damaged, the heart can still function.

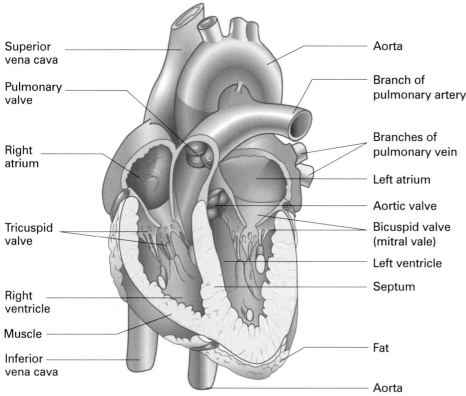

Figure 2.31 Structure of the heart

Labels (left): Superior vena cava, Pulmonary valve, Right atrium, Tricuspid valve, Right ventricle, Muscle, Inferior vena cava

Labels (right): Aorta, Branch of pulmonary artery, Branches of pulmonary vein, Left atrium, Aortic valve, Bicuspid valve (mitral vale), Left ventricle, Septum, Fat, Aorta

The atria are the top (collecting) chambers and the ventricles are the bottom (pumping) chambers. The right-hand side receives deoxygenated blood (blood without oxygen and pumps it into the lungs), and the left-hand side of the heart receives oxygenated blood (blood carrying oxygen) from the lungs and pumps it around the body.

Functions of the heart

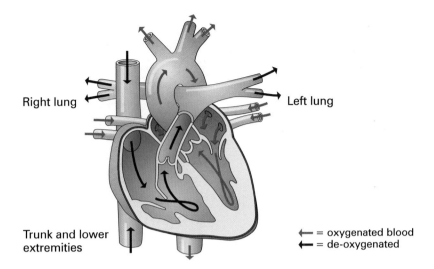

Right lung

Left lung

Trunk and lower
extremities

⟵ = oxygenated blood
⟵ = de-oxygenated

Figure 2.32 *The path of blood through the heart*

Effects of exercise on the heart

The average adult heart beats approximately 60–80 times per minute during rest and this rate increases during exercise. Any change from a resting state will cause a slight increase in heart rate.

Fitness levels can be identified by measuring resting heart rate. However, many factors must be taken into account, such as gender, health status and lifestyle. In general, females have been found to have faster resting heart rates compared to males with a similar lifestyle and level of fitness. This may be a result of females having smaller hearts, so the heart needs to beat faster to supply the body with sufficient amounts of blood.

Blood vessels

Blood vessels are the routes through which blood travels to carry nutrients and gases to all of the many body parts. There are three main types of vessels in the body:

- arteries
- veins
- capillaries.

Arteries – these are thick and elastic in texture and carry blood away from the heart. The muscle action of these vessels pushes the blood through the arteries to the relevant parts of the body.

Veins – these vessels are two layers thick and contain pocket valves to carry blood back to the heart.

! VESSEL FACT

Damaged pocket valves can result in varicose veins.

! HEART FACT

The left ventricle is the largest chamber of the heart and the cavity of this chamber increases in size as a result of endurance training.

▶ ACTION POINT

Using your index and middle finger, take your or a partner's resting radial or carotid pulse. Perform ten press-ups and ten jumping jacks, then take the pulse immediately afterwards. Note the changes (if any).

! VESSEL FACT

The blood passes through the arteries by means of the Windkessel function: the blood is pushed when contraction occurs within the vessel.

Capillaries – the delivery of nutrients and the removal of waste products occur via the diffusion of chemicals and gases in the capillaries.

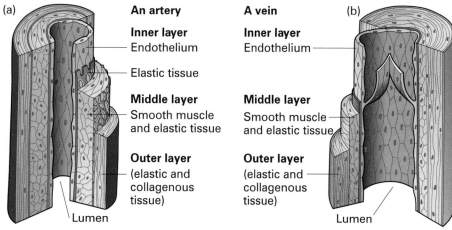

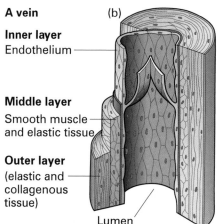

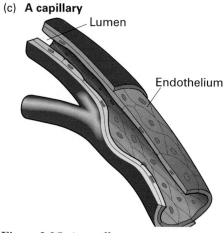

Figure 2.33 *An artery*

Figure 2.34 *A vein*

Figure 2.35 *A capillary*

The lumen is the passageway through which blood flows. The lumen in each type of blood vessel has a different diameter depending on the activity that the vessel must perform.

Blood

Types of blood cells

The total volume of blood in the body differs for individuals depending on gender, body size and fitness levels. Men on average have five to six litres of blood; women on average have four to five litres.

The blood is made up of 55 per cent plasma and 45 per cent blood cells. There are three types of blood cell: red blood cells (erythrocytes), white blood cells (leukocytes), and platelets (thrombocytes).

Plasma

Plasma is a watery liquid. It is pale yellow in colour and contains substances such as salts and calcium, nutrients (including glucose), hormones, carbon dioxide and other waste from body cells.

Red blood cells

Red blood cells are formed in the red marrow of the long bones, sternum, ribs and vertebrae. These give blood its colour and contain haemoglobin, which carries oxygen from the lungs to all the body cells. These cells have a very short lifespan of 120 days.

Platelets

Platelets are formed in the bone marrow. These cells stick together very easily and produce clots when vessels are damaged.

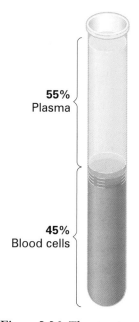

Figure 2.36 *The structure of blood*

! **BLOOD FACT**

Leukaemia (a disease of the blood) occurs as a result of abnormal white blood cells in the bone marrow.

White blood cells

White blood cells are formed in the bone marrow, lymph nodes and spleen. There are fewer of these cells compared to the red blood cells, and the white blood cells are three times the size of red blood cells. The function of these cells is to deal with fighting infections and disease. Some of these cells eat the germs that cause infection and others produce antibodies to destroy germs.

MASSAGE POINT

Massage usually helps the flow of blood back to the heart. The smaller veins (venules) that feed into the larger veins lie very close to the skin's surface and the slight pressure of an effleurage technique can help further by directing the blood to the heart. Massage can also increase the removal of waste products and toxins into the blood stream. Speeding this process up can also increase the circulation of oxygen and other nutrients around the body.

As a post-event consideration, the capillaries found in the surface of the skin respond to gentle stroking techniques that help to cool the body.

CONTRAINDICATIONS TO MASSAGE

- ☐ Do not massage over varicose veins.
- ☐ Do not massage if your client has a history of thrombosis (blood clot) or deep vein thrombosis.
- ☐ Do not massage if blood pressure is dangerously high or low – refer to a doctor.
- ☐ Do not massage if the client has a history of phlebitis (inflammation of the walls of veins).

KEYWORDS

You should now be able to define the following keywords.

arteries	deoxygenated blood	veins
atria	leukaemia	ventricles
capillaries	oxygenated blood	Windkessel function
cardiac muscle	platelets	

! BLOOD FACT

Vitamin K is a nutrient that helps to clot blood.

! BLOOD FACT

Blood pressure is the force exerted by the blood against the blood vessels.

▶ **KNOWLEDGE CHECK**

1 What is the muscle tissue of the heart called?

2 Name the three tissue layers of the heart.

3 List the four chambers of the heart.

4 What type of vessel is the aorta?

5 What is the main function of veins?

6 What effect does endurance training have on the heart?

7 Which components make up approximately 45 per cent of blood?

8 What is the primary function of white blood cells?

9 What is the average resting heart rate for an adult?

10 Name two benefits of massage on the cardiovascular system.

The respiratory system

The respiratory system helps the body to take in oxygen and remove carbon dioxide and heat from the body.

What you will learn about

- ☐ The structure of the respiratory system
- ☐ The function of the respiratory system
- ☐ Exercise and the respiratory system

The structure of the respiratory system

The respiratory system is the breathing machine of the body. It includes the mouth, nose, larynx (voice box), trachea (windpipe), lungs, diaphragm, intercostal muscles, and the thoracic cage (ribcage).

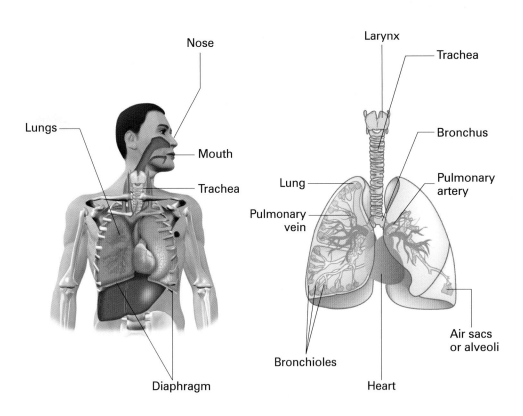

Figure 2.37 *The respiratory system*

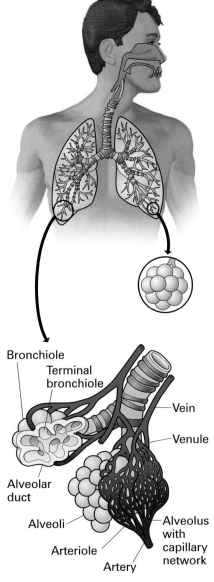

Figure 2.38 *The structure of the lungs*

Oxygen comes in through the nose and mouth and travels down the trachea until it arrives at the bronchi, which direct the air into the right lung and the left lung. The bronchi are divided further into smaller branches known as bronchioles, which have small air sacs (alveoli) at the tips to allow oxygen and other nutrients to change places.

The capillaries surrounding the alveoli collect oxygen, carrying this and other nutrients via the heart and blood circulation to all the cells of the body. Carbon dioxide and other waste products are removed from the cells by the blood, which carries them back, via the heart, to the alveoli in the lungs for exit on the out breath.

The function of the respiratory system

The respiratory system allows the passage of oxygen through the body and the removal of waste products. The diaphragm and the intercostal muscles help with the process of breathing. The diaphragm is situated below the lungs and contracts and flattens when we breathe in (inspiration). When we breathe in the intercostal muscles lift and expand the thoracic cage to allow the lungs to fill up with air, which contains oxygen. When we breathe out (expiration), the diaphragm and the intercostal muscles relax and the lungs deflate.

During the process of breathing in and out, an exchange of gases occurs. Oxygen is breathed in and moves to the alveoli and then through the tissues into the blood to supply the body via the heart. Carbon dioxide is carried in the blood as it travels from the heart to the lungs. This blood moves across into the alveoli tissue to be removed when the body breathes out.

Exercise and the respiratory system

Respiratory frequency or breathing rate is the number of breaths taken in and out per minute. The number of breaths depends on several factors including age, fitness level, lifestyle and gender. Respiratory frequency can double or triple during high intensity work. This increase during exercise is due to an increase in oxygen demand from the working muscles and a build-up of waste products such as carbon dioxide. An increase in respiratory frequency helps to satisfy oxygen demands and lowers the increasing levels of carbon dioxide and lactic acid.

> ▶ ACTION POINT
>
> As you breathe in and out, identify the body parts that move.

! RESPIRATORY FACT

An average adult breathes in and out sixteen times per minute. This is known as his or her respiratory frequency.

▶ ACTION POINT

1 With a partner, count the number of breaths that each of you takes in and out for one minute. Ensure that if you are the one being tested, you are sitting on a chair with a back rest and you are also relaxed.

2 Compare these resting values with breaths recorded after exercising for approximately five minutes. You may wish to use a combination of different exercises such as sprinting on the spot, jumping jacks and squat thrusts.

! RESPIRATORY FACT

The lungs contain small air sacs called alveoli. Their surface area is the size of a tennis court.

MASSAGE POINT

Massage can help the muscles that are involved in the respiratory system work. The respiratory system includes the thoracic cage (ribcage), the lungs and various muscles that assist in breathing. Massage can help strengthen the muscles of the thorax and the diaphragm, making these muscle groups more efficient.

Some massage techniques such as percussion can be used to increase the elastic property of muscles and circulation of blood and nutrients to the tissues. Massage can indirectly increase the volume of air that is breathed in and out per breath. This is due to an increase in the oxygen made available during breathing and helps with the exchange of this oxygen with the carbon dioxide that needs to be removed.

CONTRAINDICATIONS TO MASSAGE

- ☐ Do not massage if your client is feeling unwell.
- ☐ Do not massage if your client is suffering from a bad dose of flu or has a bad cold.

KEYWORDS

You should now be able to define the following keywords.

alveoli	larynx	respiratory system
diaphragm	lungs	thoracic cage
intercostal muscles	respiratory frequency	trachea

▶ KNOWLEDGE CHECK

1 List the structures that make up the respiratory system.

2 Name the muscles that assist in breathing.

3 What are the air sacs that are found in the lungs called?

4 Describe what happens to the thoracic cage during inspiration.

5 Describe what happens to the thoracic cage during expiration.

6 Define respiratory frequency.

7 Give two reasons why breathing rate increases during exercise.

8 Explain the benefits of sports massage to the respiratory system.

The skin

The skin is the largest organ of the body and can be described as a waterproof overcoat that fits a person whatever size they are. The skin is very flexible and can contract and expand when necessary. The skin also has the ability to repair itself once it has been damaged (e.g. by cuts or burns). This resilient cover also helps to maintain the shape of the body and to keep the internal elements inside. The skin contains sweat and oil glands that, together with its firm but flexible qualities, enable the body to move very easily.

What you will learn about

- Structure of the skin
- Skin colour
- Function of the skin

Structure of the skin

There are three layers that make up the skin:

- epidermis
- dermis
- hypodermis (often termed as the fatty layer of the skin).

> **! SKIN FACT**
>
> Most house dust is made up of dead skin.

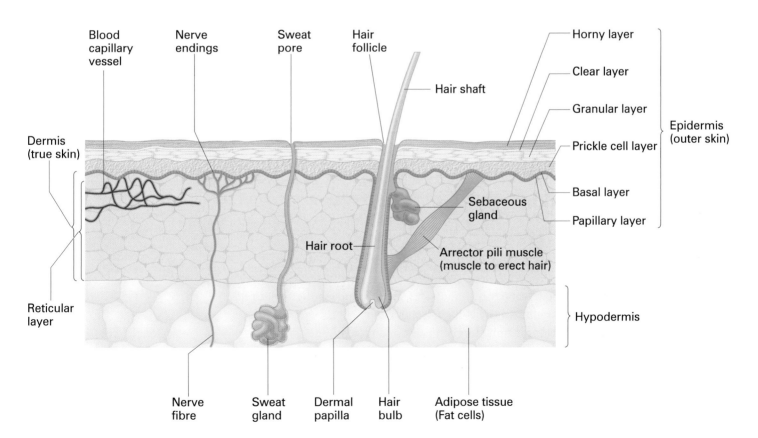

Figure 2.39 *The skin*

Epidermis

This is the top layer, which is needed for protection. It is made up of flat and dead cells. The epidemis' primary function is the protection of the body. It is attached to the next layer, which is called the dermis.

Dermis

The elastic fibres of this middle layer of the skin help it to expand and contract, giving it its elastic consistency. The blood vessels that supply the dermis feed the skin with food and oxygen. The nerve endings that are found in the dermis send messages to the central nervous system about what the skin feels and experiences: that is, cold, warmth, pain or pressure.

This second layer of the skin also contains hair follicles, which produce the hairs on the surface of the skin. Each hair stands on end or lies down by means of the arrector pili muscle that controls the hair. Adjacent to the hair, sebaceous glands produce oil (sebum), which maintains the flexibility of the skin and helps to produce an acid substance to protect the skin from germs. The dermis also contains the sweat glands, which help the surface of the skin to stay cool, especially during exercise or exposure to hot environmental conditions.

Hypodermis

The hypodermis, the third layer, is found under the dermis. This layer contains adipose tissue (fat), which facilitates maintenance of warmth and gives protection. This adipose tissue also acts as an energy store for the body. It is this third layer that is the link between the skin and the inside of the body; that is, the musculoskeletal system.

Skin colour

The skin contains a protein called melanin, which gives the skin its colour. High levels of melanin result in the skin having a darker tone; a lower level gives the skin a fairer colour. When exposed to the sun's rays, an increase in the production of melanin occurs, giving the skin a 'tan'.

Functions of the skin

The skin has many functions. The key functions are listed below:

- **Protection** – skin protects us from some harmful poisons or chemicals, diseases and ultraviolet rays.
- **Maintains body temperature** – As body heat increases, sweat glands in the skin help to cool the body by releasing sweat that then evaporates.
- **Produces vitamin D** – this helps in bone formation and maintenance.
- **Protects fat stores** – as the skin grows, the fat stores underneath the skin increase. This helps in the protection and temperature regulation of the body.
- **Releases waste products** – carbon dioxide and other waste products are released through perspiration.
- **Moisturises** – the sebaceous glands release a natural, oily, moisturising lubricant called sebum onto the skin surface. This helps to protect the skin from harmful bacteria.

> **! SKIN FACT**
>
> High exposure to the sun's rays can increase the risk of skin cancer; however, normal day-to-day exposure helps to maintain levels of vitamin D. While this is true, sun protection is still necessary.

☐ **Sensitivity** – the skin contains many nerve endings, which allow the perception of cold, heat, pain and pressure. The skin has an extensive nerve supply that informs the body about the environment. The cells that are part of the nervous system are found towards the top of the dermis and are sensitive to cold, light, pain and pressure. Greater pressures are sensed by receptors that are found deeper in the dermis. There are more pain receptors in the skin than receptors that detect changes in body temperature.

MASSAGE POINT

Massage helps many of the body's systems to function more efficiently by increasing the flow of blood. It also helps in the production of sebum, which helps to make the skin softer and more supple.

Massage can act as a buffer to clear away dead cells from the top layer of the skin. This helps the skin to breathe more freely and is known as desquamation.

CONTRAINDICATIONS: THE SKIN

☐ Do not massage over any infectious skin disease, for example, impetigo.
☐ Do not massage over any open cuts, wounds, breaks in the skin surface, or fresh bruising.
☐ Do not massage over warts or moles.

! SKIN FACT

Pores allow the skin to breathe. The skin also possesses tiny hairs that grow all over the body except the soles of the feet and palms of the hands.

KEYWORDS

You should now be able to define the following keywords.

adipose tissue

hypodermis

sebum

dermis

melanin

epidermis

perspiration

▶ KNOWLEDGE CHECK

1 Name the three layers that make up the skin.
2 Give the correct term for the layer of fat stored under the skin.
3 Name the chemical substance that provides the skin with a natural moisturiser.
4 What gives the skin its colour?
5 Name five functions of the skin.
6 What is the skin at risk of if exposed to high levels of the sun's rays?
7 Which vitamin does the sun supply to the skin?
8 Which layer of the skin contains the sweat glands?
9 What do pores allow the skin to do?
10 Which gland secretes sebum?

The nervous system

The nervous system is the control mechanism of the human body. It controls all of the functions of the human body by working in partnership with the endocrine system, sending and receiving messages to affect other systems and their functions.

What you will learn about

☐ Structure of the nervous system

☐ Nerve cell structure

☐ Function of the nervous system

Structure of the nervous system

The nervous system is divided into two sections:

1 the central nervous system (CNS)

2 the peripheral nervous system (PNS).

The central nervous system is made up of the brain and the spinal cord. It is connected to the rest of the body via the peripheral nervous system (PNS). This is made up of the spinal and cranial nerves, which continuously send messages to the CNS for processing before returning them to the PNS.

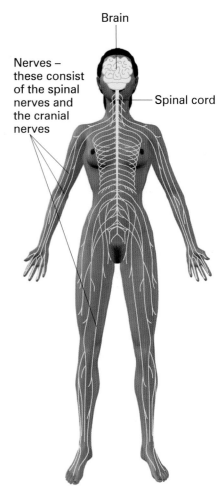

Figure 2.40 *The nervous system*

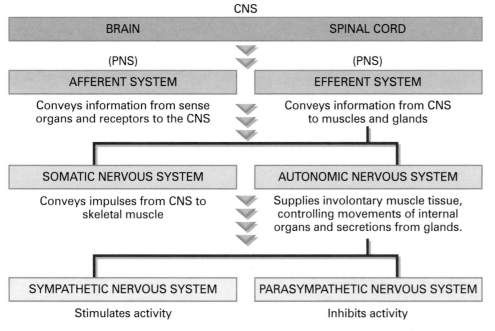

Figure 2.41 *The organization of the central nervous system*

The PNS is divided into three elements: the motor, sensory and autonomic systems.

☐ The motor nerves carry information from the brain to the muscles that are used for movement.

☐ The sensory nerves transmit information to the CNS.

☐ The autonomic nerves are responsible for controlling the functions of the vital organs and glands in the body.

The autonomic nervous system is subdivided into sympathetic and parasympathetic nervous system. Both systems are involved in regulating bodily functions. In a stressful situation, the autonomic nervous system causes physiological changes, such as:

- increase in heart rate
- increase in blood pressure
- dilation of blood vessels
- dilation of pupils of the eyes
- increase in the production of glucose in the liver
- increase in the production of sweat.

These changes help to prepare the body for the stressful situation. Once the stressful situation has passed, the parasympathetic nerves should take over and help the body to return to its normal state.

Some nerves are bundled together in fascicles. These fascicles consist of two different types of fibres: afferent and efferent fibres. The afferent fibres carry information from the receptors of the skin, sensory organs and vital organs to the brain and the spinal cord (CNS). The efferent fibres carry information from the CNS to the muscle or gland that the body needs to move or activate.

Nerve cell structure

A single cell of the nervous system is called a neurone or nerve cell. A neurone is made up of a cell body, an axon (or nerve fibre) and dendrites. The axon and dendrites of the neurone run from the cell body; the axon is covered by a myelin sheath. The axon carries nerve impulses away from the cell and the dendrites receive signals from other cells or neurons.

Function of the nervous system

The brain and spinal cord work together to control and co-ordinate the movements of the rest of the body.

> **! NERVE FACT**
>
> The transmission of nerve impulses increases due to the myelin sheath found around the axon.

> **! NERVE FACT**
>
> Some axons or nerve fibres are as long as one metre.

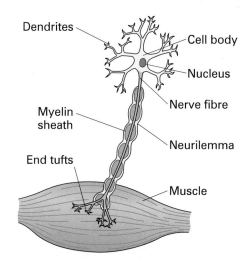

Figure 2.41 A *motor neurone*

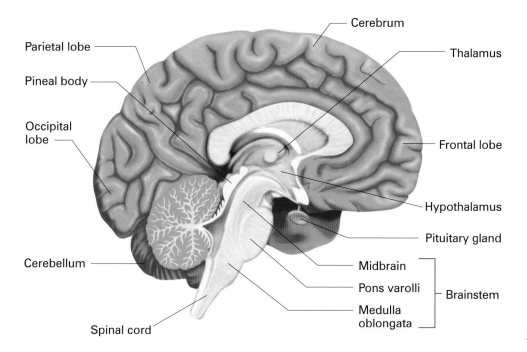

Figure 2.42 *The brain*

The largest section of the brain is the cerebrum. This can be divided into four lobes: the frontal, temporal, occipital and parietal lobes. The brain is also divided into left and right by a deep groove in the cerebrum called the longitudinal fissure. This contains a network of nerves that constantly communicate with each other.

The cerebellum helps to control balance and posture, and is the link between the brain and the spinal cord. The spinal cord is a cable approximately 43cm in length. It is divided into two sections – grey matter that contains inner structures of the cord and white matter, which forms the outer layer.

The inner grey matter contains nerve cells without myelin sheaths. These cells aid in protection and transmission. The white matter contains axons with a myelin sheath to increase the speed of impulses travelling between the brain and the spinal cord.

The brain contains cranial nerves that link the CNS to the PNS. There are twelve pairs of these nerves, usually found in the head and neck area. Some possess fibres from the sensory and the motor fibre group. These give information to the brain about the tension of muscle and the balance of the body.

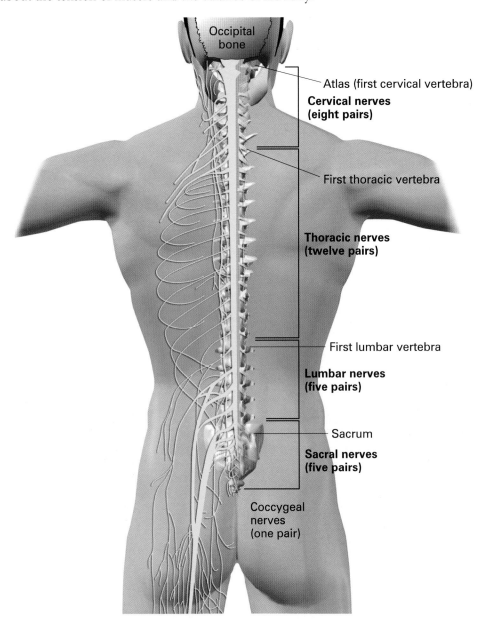

Figure 2.43 *The spinal nerves*

Occipital bone

Atlas (first cervical vertebra)
Cervical nerves (eight pairs)

First thoracic vertebra

Thoracic nerves (twelve pairs)

First lumbar vertebra

Lumbar nerves (five pairs)

Sacrum

Sacral nerves (five pairs)

Coccygeal nerves (one pair)

The vertebral column forms the skeletal protection for the spinal cord. Further protection is provided by cerebrospinal fluid, which circulates the outer brain as well as the length of the spinal cord.

31 pairs of spinal nerves rise from the spinal cord, emerging from the gaps between the vertebrae to travel through the tissues to every part of the body. These provide the communication system between the brain and those body parts. For example, the pain sensation from straining a muscle is transmitted via these nerves back to the spinal cord and the brain. A return instruction might be to stop the activity which caused the strain.

MASSAGE POINT

Massage techniques such as vibrations, frictions and percussion can stimulate nerves of the body. Placing slight pressure on the nerves can also block impulses, providing temporary relief from pain by causing a numbing or deadening sensation in the area.

Slow, smooth movements can also produce a relaxing sensation in specific areas. Movements that are slow, but not too deep and rhythmical, can increase the relaxation effect on the nerves. This may result in your client falling asleep, but he or she will wake up feeling refreshed. However, some massage techniques around the head and back areas can also have a beneficial effect on the central nervous system.

KEYWORDS

You should now be able to define the following keywords.

brain

cranial nerves

spinal cord

central nervous system

peripheral nervous system

CONTRAINDICATIONS TO MASSAGE

☐ Do not massage any muscle spasticity.
☐ Do not massage an individual who has uncontrolled epilepsy (someone who is not taking any medication for this condition).

▶ KNOWLEDGE CHECK

1 Name the two parts that make up the central nervous system.
2 What are sensory nerves responsible for?
3 Describe how the efferent nerves work.
4 What skeletal structure protects the spinal cord?
5 Label the diagram of a neurone.
6 What is the largest section of the brain?
7 What is the purpose of the sensory nerves?
8 What type of massage technique can benefit the nervous system?

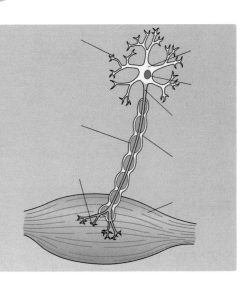

The endocrine system

The main purpose of the endocrine system is to maintain a balance of the environment within the human body through the release of hormones.

What you will learn about

□ How the endocrine system works
□ Function of the endocrine system

How the endocrine system works

The 'chemical signals' that the body sends to the different parts of the body are known as hormones. The hormones that are released come from endocrine glands found in various parts of the body. Each gland secretes specific hormones with specific roles to carry out. For example, the pituitary gland releases the growth hormone somatotrophin, which controls general growth in the body, and gonadotrophins, which control the maturation of eggs in the ovaries and the production of sperm in the testes.

The endocrine glands secrete hormones directly into the blood, which carries them to the target cells, which may be far from the area of secretion. Hormone receptors in the target cells receive only the hormones relevant to the cells' function.

Function of the endocrine system

The endocrine system is responsible for:

□ regulating the chemical make-up of the body
□ regulating body metabolism and energy balance
□ ensuring that the immune system functions correctly
□ controlling the factors that help smooth muscle and cardiac muscle contact.

Production site	Hormones
pancreas	insulin
adrenal cortex	cortisol and aldosterone
ovaries	oestrogen and progesterone
testes	testosterone
placenta	oestrogen and progesterone
adrenal gland	epinephrine and norepiphrine
thyroid gland	thyroxine and triiodothyronine

Figure 2.44 The production sites of hormones

The pituitary gland

This gland is situated at the base of the brain and is often called the master gland because its hormones help to control so many of the other endocrine glands in the body. However, it is known that the **hypothalamus** produces secretions that regulate the pituitary gland. The gland has two parts, the anterior and the posterior lobes.

The anterior lobe produces the following hormones:

Hormone	Action/effect
• Thyroid stimulating hormone (TSH)	Controls the thyroid gland
• Adrenocorticotrophic hormone (ACTH)	Stimulates the adrenal cortex
• Somatotrophin or growth hormone (GH)	Controls general body growth
• Follicle stimulating hormone (FSH)	Stimulates the production of eggs in the ovaries and sperm in the testes
• Luteinising hormone (LH)	Prepares the uterus for implantation of the egg and prepares the mammary glands for milk production in the female. In the male it stimulates the testes to develop and secrete testosterone.
• Prolactin (PRL)	Initiates and maintains milk secretion

The posterior lobe stores the following hormones produced by the hypothalamus:

Hormone	Action/effect
• Vasopressin antdiuretic hormone (ADH)	Decreases urine volume
• Oxytocin	Stimulates the uterus to contract and the mammary glands to produce milk

! HORMONE FACT

Hormones and their target cells work within a 'lock-and-key' system. The lock is the target cell and the hormone is the key. Only the correct key (hormone) can open the lock (target cell).

MASSAGE POINT

Sports massage helps to relieve stress and supports the endocrine system in maintaining body homeostasis (internal equilibrium). Stress affects the body in different ways. Your client may suffer from headaches, chest pains or breathlessness, amongst other symptoms.

KEYWORDS

You should now be able to define the following keywords.

hormones

target cells

CONTRAINDICATIONS TO MASSAGE

☐ Massage can be applied to a client suffering from diabetes. However, it is important to be aware of any medication that is being taken and to inform him or her that massage may alter glucose levels.

☐ If you are unsure about the situation, seek medical advice or request a referral letter from your client's GP.

▶ KNOWLEDGE CHECK

1 What are the 'chemical signals' that the endocrine system releases called?

2 Give two examples of glands that release 'chemical signals'.

3 Which gland is responsible for releasing the growth hormone somatotrophin?

4 List the four functions of the endocrine system.

The lymphatic system

The lymphatic system consists of a network of fine vessels found throughout the body except in bone tissue, cartilage, the central nervous system and the teeth. The vessels collect excess fluids from the body tissues, filtering it through clusters of small, round structures called nodes. The fluid travelling in the lymph vessels (now known as lymph) finally returns to the blood via ducts entering the large veins for circulation to the heart and lungs.

What you will learn about

☐ Structure of the lymphatic system
☐ Function of the lymphatic system

Structure of the lymphatic system

The lymphatic system is made up of the following structures:

☐ Lymphatic capillaries collect lymph from surrounding tissues.
☐ Lymphatic vessels transport lymph. They contain valves which ensure that the lymph travels in the right direction. These valves give the vessels a 'pearl necklace' appearance when the vessels are full.

> **! LYMPHATIC FACT**
>
> Lymph is clear or straw-coloured.

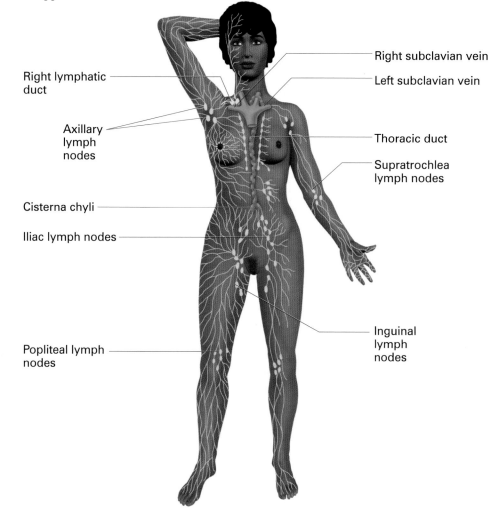

Right subclavian vein
Left subclavian vein
Right lymphatic duct
Axillary lymph nodes
Thoracic duct
Supratrochlea lymph nodes
Cisterna chyli
Iliac lymph nodes
Inguinal lymph nodes
Popliteal lymph nodes

Figure 2.45 The lymphatic system

- Lymph nodes are flat, round and approximately the size of a kidney bean. They are found in clusters around the body, for example, behind the knees, in the armpits and under the jawline. The largest nodes are found in the neck region. The nodes filter bacteria and debris from the lymph as it passes through. Each node is 97 per cent blood plasma and three per cent solid parts.

- The two lymph ducts, the right lymphatic duct and the thoracic duct, drain lymph from the body and empty it into the venous system.

! LYMPHATIC FACT

The fluid found in the intestinal lymph vessels is known as chyle.

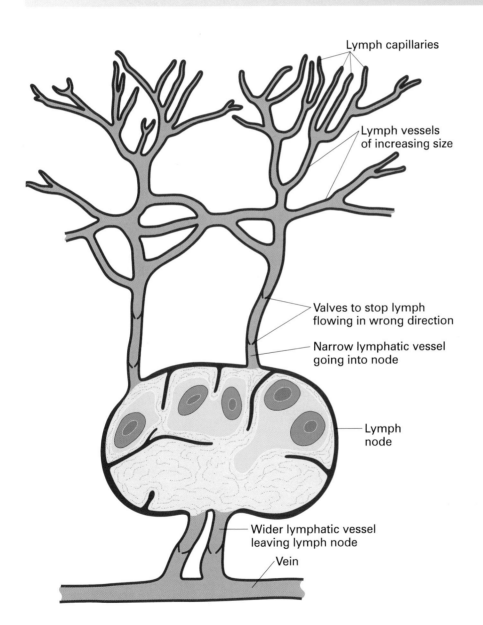

Figure 2.46 Lymph node

Lymph capillaries

Lymph vessels of increasing size

Valves to stop lymph flowing in wrong direction

Narrow lymphatic vessel going into node

Lymph node

Wider lymphatic vessel leaving lymph node

Vein

! LYMPHATIC FACT

There are between 400 and 600 lymph nodes in the human body.

During the diffusion of gases in the blood capillaries, some of the blood plasma filters from the capillaries into the tissues. This is called interstitial fluid or tissue fluid. Most of this fluid returns to the blood capillaries after the exchange of gases; the fluid that is left is known as lymph.

Blood and lymph transport various substances between cells:

- Flowing lymph – runs through the lymphatic system
- Interstitial lymph – where all cells bathe in the intercellular lymph.

The cells of the body swim in a sea of fluid. However, only eight litres are needed for the cells to survive in the body; therefore, the cells are quite tightly compacted in their environment.

- 60–70 per cent of body weight is water.
- Two-thirds of this water is inside the cells.
- One-third of this water is found in blood.

This system is very important in maintaining the fluid balance in the tissues and ensuring that the interstitial fluid is returned to the blood to maintain the correct balance.

Function of the lymphatic system

There are three main functions of the lymphatic system:

1   to collect lymph from the body tissues

2   to collect digested fats in the intestines for further circulation. When fats are present in the lymphatic fluid it appears cloudy and is called chyle.

3   to develop lymphocytes in the lymph nodes. Lymphocytes defend the body against harmful bacteria that could cause infection. They are the second line of defence against bacteria after antibodies, which are produced by some white blood cells.

MASSAGE POINT

Various massage techniques can improve the circulation of fluid in the body. Effleurage and kneading aids the lymphatic system by helping to release lymph and enabling it to travel more easily to specific node clusters.

Care must be taken to identify problem areas that need to be avoided in massage. However, massage can be of benefit when lymphatic vessels become blocked and swollen due to waste not being moved and removed.

KEYWORDS

You should now be able to define the following keywords.

chyle   lymph

duct   lymph nodes

interstitial fluid

tissue fluid

▶ KNOWLEDGE CHECK

1 Describe the role of the lymphatic system.

2 Where in the body are there no lymphatic structures?

3 What is the role of lymph nodes?

4 How many lymph nodes are there in the human body?

5 What is the role of chyle?

6 Name the four types of lymphatic structures.

7 Where can lymphocytes be found?

8 What is the primary role of lymphocytes?

9 What is the primary role of lymphatic vessels?

10 How does sports massage benefit the lymphatic system?

You the
professional

Code of ethics

All of the governing bodies and professional associations involved in sports massage and sports therapy set rules which should be followed in order to maintain good practice. These rules are referred to as a code of ethics or code of practice. Upon becoming a member of an association, such as the International Institute of Sports Therapy (IIST), the therapist must agree to abide by the code of ethics laid down by the professional body. A code of ethics is put in place to ensure that all therapists:

- provide a professional service
- work to a standard which is laid down by the associations
- abide by all rules and regulations relating to health, safety and hygiene
- follow correct procedures and work within the limits of training and qualifications
- practise with adequate insurance cover.

It is essential that you adhere to certain standards in order to maintain good practice. For example:

- you should behave in a professional manner at all times
- you must maintain client confidentiality
- where contraindications have been identified, or if your client is under medical supervision, you should ask your client to provide written consent from his or her doctor before commencing treatment
- you must not try to diagnose medical conditions or give treatment or advice that is beyond the scope of your training
- you must show respect to other practitioners.

Whilst studying for a qualification in sports massage, you will be eligible to join relevant associations as a student member and may receive a number of benefits including:

- reduced fees upon becoming a full member
- student insurance cover
- codes of practice for the industry
- a members' catalogue for the purchase of products for massage therapy.

Upon qualifying you will be eligible to join as a full member and have access to the following benefits:

- full member insurance cover
- a monthly newsletter containing relevant information on therapy issues
- an update on any changes in the law
- discounts from equipment suppliers
- access to free helplines for queries
- an application to be listed on the National Register of Therapists.

▶ **ACTION POINT**

1 Using magazines such as *The Therapist*, recent issues of health and safety journals, newspaper articles, and so on, find two different examples from the health, fitness, holistic or sports therapy industry where a code of ethics, health and safety rules or regulations have not been followed.

2 Discuss your findings in small groups and answer the following questions.

a What happened to all of the people involved, for example, the therapist, client, and so on?

b What code of ethics, rule or regulation was breached?

c What measures could have been taken to avoid any incident/ accident that may have happened?

d What could the cost be to a business and a professional therapist for failing to implement safe working practices?

Personal and professional presentation

As a sports massage therapist, it is essential that the first impression you give is the one that you want your clients to remember you by. As a professional, it is important that you *are* professional and that you follow all of the dos and don'ts shown below.

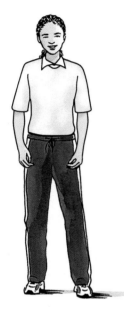 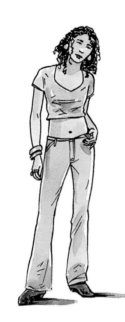

DO

- ☐ Tie your hair back and keep it away from your face.
- ☐ Keep your nails clean and short. Avoid wearing nail varnish.
- ☐ Wear clean trainers, tracksuit bottoms and a polo shirt or regulated uniform (if provided).
- ☐ Wash, and use an anti-perspirant to eliminate body odour.
- ☐ Wear appropriate footwear to encourage comfort for a full day's work and for safety of movement when dealing with your client.
- ☐ Ensure that oral care has been maintained to avoid bad breath and tooth decay.

DON'T

- ☐ Allow your hair to fall over your face.
- ☐ Varnish nails or have long, chipped nails; this gives an impression of a lack of self-care.
- ☐ Wear jewellery.
- ☐ Wear tight clothing that stops you from moving freely when massaging your client.
- ☐ Wear heavy or stale make-up.
- ☐ Smother yourself with strong perfume.

Figure 3.1 Dos and don'ts of professional presentation

It is vital to look professional and act professionally from the first day of training and this approach should be maintained throughout your working life. Remember that you do not get a second chance to make a first impression.

Your business

As a therapist dealing with the public, you need to protect your business, your clients and yourself. You will need to be aware of and abide by the appropriate regulations and legislation in order to maintain health and safety within the working environment. You also need to ensure the health, safety and welfare of yourself, staff and customers.

Whether your business is large or small, it will be governed by certain government regulations, Acts of Parliament and EU (European Union) Directives. It is the responsibility of the employer or clinic owner, if setting up in private practice, to obtain updated information on any changes in regulations. This will ensure that all employees, visitors and customers will be safe within the environment. Breaking the law by ignoring or not updating this information could result in severe punishment, which in turn could be costly to your business in a number of ways.

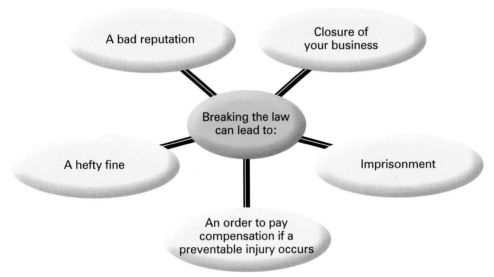

Figure 3.2 *The cost of breaking the law*

The list below shows the key legislation and regulations that you need to be aware of in order to comply with the law.

Health and Safety at Work Act 1974

Under the Health and Safety at Work Act, all employers have a duty of care to ensure that a safe working environment is provided for the health, safety and welfare of all employees. Employees also have a duty of care to ensure that their own health and safety at work and that of others – customers or visitors – is not put at risk, by complying with correct procedures. If any solutions or chemicals are used within the clinic, then these must be stored correctly and there must be information available on these in the case of an emergency. A written health and safety policy must also be available.

Manual Handling Operation Regulations 1992

Under these regulations, all staff should be trained in the correct procedures for lifting in order to prevent injuries to themselves and others. Musculo-skeletal disorders are usually a result of incorrect lifting.

Control of Substances Hazardous to Health Regulations (COSHH) 2002

Hazardous substances must be carefully controlled and stored in order to prevent harm to others. These may include chemicals that are used to sterilize equipment.

Gas Safety (Installation and Use) Regulations 1994

These regulations state that gas appliances must be regularly maintained.

Electricity at Work Regulations 1989

These regulations are concerned with safety in the use of electricity. All electrical equipment must be maintained and checked regularly. All checks, dates, times and any action taken should be noted.

Fire Precaution Workplace Regulations 1997

Fire risk assessments must be carried out at all premises and must be recorded in writing. The therapist must be aware of fire and evacuation procedures and must have knowledge, and adequate training, in a range of fire containment equipment, for use on electrical and non-electrical fires, as well as in other relevant equipment, such as fire blankets.

Reporting of Injuries, Diseases and Dangerous Occurrences Regulations (RIDDOR) 1995

Accidents and ill health must be reported and records must be kept of any accidents that occur. The following information should be included in an accident report:

- date, time and place of accident
- name, address and telephone number of those involved
- a description of what happened
- any witness details.

Diseases such as hepatitis and contagious skin infections should be reported immediately to a supervisor.

Employer's Liability (Compulsory Insurance) Act 1969

Under this Act, all employers must take out an approved insurance, which covers them for treatments and insures against liability for bodily injuries, illness or disease. The certificate of insurance must be displayed at the place of business.

The Consumer Protection Act 1987

Under this Act, all organizations must advertise or describe their products honestly and price indications should not be misleading. If your brochure states that a back massage costs £15, then you cannot charge the customer £20 at the end of the service. A customer has the right to complain to Trading Standards if something like this happens.

Health and Safety (First Aid) Regulations 1981

These regulations state that all organizations must have qualified first-aiders or appointed first-aiders who can be called upon to deal with any injuries that may occur within the organization. A fully stocked first-aid kit must also be available at all times.

Trade Descriptions Act 1968 and 1987

This Act protects the customer from being misled about products or services, as well as price indications.

Data Protection Act 1998

All information that you have about your client must be kept strictly confidential and securely stored on a computer or in a lockable filing cabinet. Information cannot be disclosed to any third party without the permission of your client. Under this Act, customers have the right to know if a company or organization holds information about them on their database. However, for a company to be able to hold customer information, they must be registered with the Data Protection Registrar.

Systems must be put in place in the workplace so that safe practice can be carried out in all areas of work. There are many responsibilities (see figure 3.3 below) and these are carried out by your employer and you the therapist if you work for someone else, and by you the therapist if you are self-employed.

Figure 3.3 Employer's responsibilities

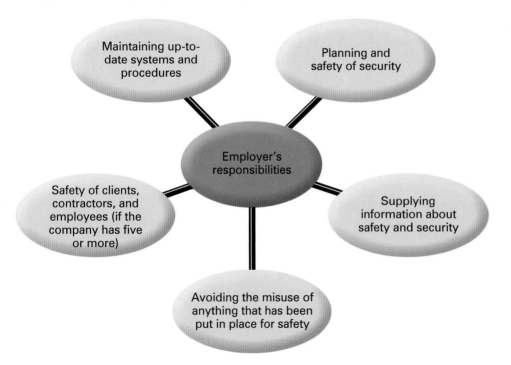

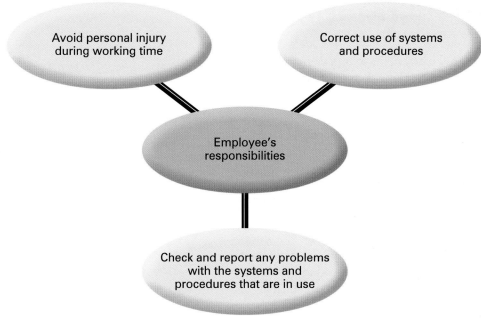

Figure 3.4 *Employee's responsibilities*

Responsibilities shared between the employer and employee include ensuring the safety of the working environment. Reasonable care in working practices should be taken by you the therapist when dealing with clients and in order to co-operate with employers in ensuring safe practice; for example, carrying out the requirements under the Health and Safety at Work Act.

Insurance

Insurance is vital when providing treatment for internal or external clients. Whether you are just starting to build a client list, or have a client base of hundreds of people, you will need insurance. Insurance provides you with protection as long as you have followed all of the necessary steps in providing a safe service within a safe working environment.

The professional body you join once you are qualified, such as the FHT (Federation of Holistic Therapies), will usually provide you with details of insurance and can offer you deals as a member. If you have people working for you, it will be necessary to provide cover for these individuals during their time at work, especially those that work with clients. Public liability insurance can protect you and your staff from claims from clients and cover can be taken out for up to £6 million.

The different types of insurance include:

□ public and treatment liability insurance
□ business equipment/employer's liability insurance
□ student's liability insurance.

> **! BUSINESS FACT**
>
> Protect yourself and your clients by taking out insurance policies whether as a student or as a qualified therapist.

Creating a safe environment

The first impressions you give to your clients are based upon your personal appearance and the environment in which you are working. You must strive to maintain a high level of cleanliness and maintain the health, safety and welfare of your clients as soon as they enter your practice. This will give a good impression of your high level of professionalism and commitment to the service you provide for each client.

It is essential that the working environment is safe and free from hazards that might harm you or your clients. This may not always be down to you; for example, when you are working in the changing rooms of a soccer team before a match, kit bags and equipment may make it difficult for you to treat a player safely. After a match there may be wet and dirty kit over the floor and benches that could hinder the efficiency of your treatment. However, your clients will still need to be treated and, it is important to be able to adapt your treatment to your environment. It may be a good idea to find a different room in which to deliver treatments if the changing rooms are occupied by other players, but it is important to remember that a separate facility may not always be available.

A safe environment must also be maintained wherever you are working or whatever conditions you are working in. There may be times when you are working in extreme heat when you may have to protect yourself from the sun by using a sun block or by wearing a cap. In very cold weather, it is important that you wrap up warm, but avoid wearing too many clothes, as these may restrict you from running across the pitch if someone is injured.

Risk Assessment

It is essential to carry out a risk assessment in all the environments that the therapist chooses to work in, including clinic, field, gymnasium and changing room. Risk assessments should always comply with the guidelines drawn up by the Health and Safety Executive (HSE).

A risk assessment should consist of five steps. Below is an example of a risk assessment procedure for performing a massage in a changing room.

> **! SAFE ENVIRONMENT FACT**
>
> Therapists may work in any of the following environments:
> - changing room
> - client's home
> - gym
> - private clinic
> - outdoor pitchside
>
> Whatever the environment, the therapist must always consider:
> - How much space is there to work in?
> - Is the area free from obstructions?
> - Is the floor or ground slippery?

Step 1 Identify possible hazard	Step 2 Identify who might be harmed	Step 3 Current measures in place	Step 4 Suggested additional measures to reduce risks	Step 5 Evaluate and review findings
Obstacles such as sports bags and equipment may be tripped over, resulting in an injury.	• Player receiving treatment. • Therapist giving treatment. • Other players in or entering the facility.	• Benches to place obstacles underneath. • Clothes hooks to hang sports . kit on	• Signs to inform players of risks associated with untidy kit. • Lockers for additional space and security.	Ongoing. Review 2 months from now.

Figure 3.5 *Example of a risk assessment procedure*

Client consultation

A client consultation is the initial way for you, the therapist, to build a rapport with a client and to gather information about his or her well-being and state of health. You will gather both subjective and objective information: subjective information is impressionistic information, which cannot be quantified, such as the degree of pain your client might be feeling; objective information is observable information, which can be quantified, such as the amount of swelling you can see.

The elements of consultation

The consultation has three elements:

1 verbal   **2** visual   **3** physical.

1 Verbal

The verbal element involves talking to your client and asking the questions 'How?, What?, Why?, Where? and When?'. For example, 'What sport do you play?', 'When did it happen?', 'Where do you feel there is a problem?', 'How do you feel?', 'Why sports massage?'

2 Visual

The visual element lasts throughout the consultation. It starts from when your client enters the room, since you will be able to observe straight away whether he or she has a postural problem (see Posture, pages 80–92). You can assess your client's posture in more detail later in the consultation and identify any problems. You also need to look at the 'trouble spots', such as bruising, discoloration, swelling, open cuts and wounds.

3 Physical

The physical element involves palpating the area. Palpation is a method which is used to feel the area in a specific way using the thumb or the whole hand. On palpation you may be able to feel soft tissue abnormalities such as muscle tension. During the physical stage of the consultation, the client may need to perform different activities so that the therapist can ascertain his or her range of movement at joints, and to see if any pain or limitation is felt during specific movements. Usually, the client will tell you whether they have experienced any pain during a particular movement.

> **! CONSULTATION FACT**
>
> You may need to ask your client to help with the physical element of the consultation. He or she can perform movements to help you establish the range of movement at specific joints.

It is vitally important that you keep an up-to-date record of all treatments given to each client. All information given to you by your client should be kept confidential and secure under the Data Protection Act and should not be disclosed to a third party. The purpose of a client consultation is to gather information about your client to establish his or her initial status. With this information you can then decide on the best course of treatment.

> **! CONSULTATION FACT**
>
> Do not assume! Ask questions to gather sufficient evidence to be able to make an informed judgement about your client's situation.

> **! CONSULTATION FACT**
>
> Postural problems can be the source of a variety of injuries. Many people suffer from postural problems without being aware of it. For example, lumbar lordosis, which is an inward curvature of the lumbar spine, can place a strain on the lower back.

The Central Academy of Sports Therapies
Sports massage consultation record

Personal details

Name	First name		Surname	
Address				
	Postcode			
Tel/fax/e-mail	Home no.	Work no.	Fax	E-mail
Date of birth				
Gender	Male/female			

Medical history

Name of doctor Address of surgery				
Tel				
General health status	Good	Average	Below average	Poor
Serious illnesses past and current				
Previous injuries				

Problems

Muscular
Skeletal
Circulatory
Allergies
Current medical treatment
Medication
Family medical history

Figure 3.6 Blank consultation record

Lifestyle

Marital status

Professional status

Exercise or sport

Smoker

Alcohol
consumption   Units per week

Identify the pain
or problems and
level of pain
(10 being
extremely
painful)

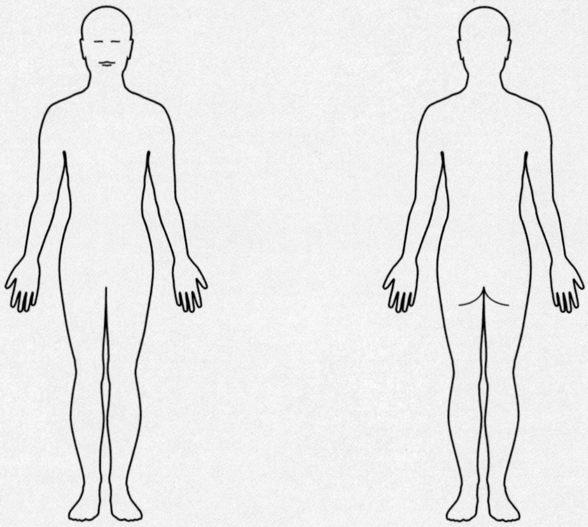

Therapist's
comments

Client signature

Therapist signature

Date

The Central Academy of Sports Therapies
Sports massage consultation record

Personal details

Name	First name	Surname
	James	*Bond*

Address   *1 Town Centre Close*
Leicester

Postcode   *LE1 2AB*

Tel/fax/e-mail	Home no.	Work no.	Fax	E-mail
	234 5678			

Date of birth   *27 October 1956*

Gender   (Male)/female

Medical history

Name of doctor   *Dr No*

Address of surgery   *Medical centre*
Leicester

Tel

General health status	(Good)	Average	Below average	Poor

Serious illnesses past and current   *Pneumonia, January 2002*

Previous injuries   *Achilles tendonitis (right)*

Problems

Muscular   *Tight right calf*

Skeletal   *N/A*

Circulatory   *N/A*

Allergies   *Nut allergy, penicillin*

Current medical treatment   *None*

Medication   *None*

Family medical history   *Father – heart attack at 58 years*

Figure 3.7 Completed consultation record

Lifestyle

Marital status	*Married*
Professional status	*Teacher*
Exercise or sport	*Cycles to work every day (eight miles round trip)* *Gym twice a week* *Running club once a week*
Smoker	*No*
Alcohol consumption	Units per week *18 units per week*

Identify the pain or problems and level of pain (10 being extremely painful)

Pain occurs before and after exercise. Pain increases during passive stretching of the area in dorsiflexion and in plantarflexion when resistance is present

Therapist's comments

Ice massage of the area; restrict sports participation for approximately three weeks. Treatments should include: mobilization of frictions of the Achilles tendon. Mobilize the ankle; and general massage of the whole area of the calf muscle. Include active stretches of the Achilles tendon during treatment sessions, before and after training.

Client signature

Therapist signature

Date

The Central Academy of Sports Therapies Sports massage consultation record				
Personal details				
Name	First name *Peter*	Surname *Parker*			
Address	*1 Spiderweb Avenue* *Leicester* Postcode *LE1 3EB*			
Tel/fax/e-mail	Home no. *987 5643*	Work no.	Fax	E-mail
Date of birth	*1 March 1965*			
Gender	(Male)/female			
Medical history				
Name of doctor	*Dr Claus*			
Address of surgery	*Royal College Hospital* *Leicester*			
Tel				
General health status	(Good)	Average	Below average	Poor
Serious illnesses past and current	*N/A*			
Previous injuries	*Right shoulder injury* *Over-extension of the right arm at the elbow joint. When this injury* *occurred, tearing sound was heard*			
Problems				
Muscular	*Pain at the elbow joint. Sometimes tingling and numbness of the* *forearm area is felt*			
Skeletal	*N/A*			
Circulatory	*N/A*			
Allergies	*None*			
Current medical treatment	*None*			
Medication	*None*			
Family medical history	*None*			

Figure 3.8 Semi-completed consultation record

▶ ACTION POINT

Complete the following sports massage consultation record by identifying the injury and the massage treatment that might be offered.

Lifestyle

Marital status	*Single*
Professional status	*Media reporter*
Exercise or sport	*Gymnastics coach*
Smoker	*No*
Alcohol consumption	Units per week *14 units per week*

Identify the pain or problems and level of pain (10 being extremely painful)

Pain at the elbow area and during overhead movements

Therapist's comments

Client signature

Therapist signature

Date

Posture

Regular participation in different sporting activities can lead to the development of muscle bulk in the side of the body or, specifically, in the areas that are continuously used in a sporting activity. It can also produce tightness within the muscle and could result in a muscle strength imbalance on either side of the body. When combined, these can lead to postural deviations, which can affect sporting performance and may lead to injuries.

Good posture is crucial not just for sports people but for everyone. Strong abdominal and back muscles will help maintain a good posture as well as a pelvic tilt. The pelvis must be in a balanced position and slightly tilted to enable the back to be at its strongest. In this position the strain placed upon the muscles is reduced.

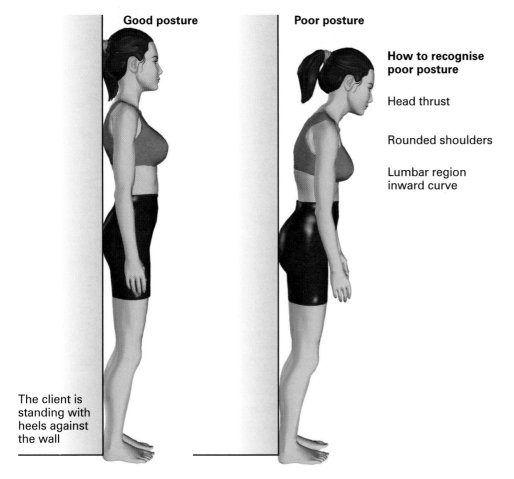

Good posture

Poor posture

How to recognise poor posture

Head thrust

Rounded shoulders

Lumbar region inward curve

The client is standing with heels against the wall

Figure 3.9 Assessment of posture

> ▶ **ACTION POINT**
>
> For all action points in this section:
> 1 State the length of time for which each exercise should be carried out.
>
> 2 State the number of repetitions that you would advise the client to do.
>
> 3 State the amount of time which a client should hold a stretch.

An athlete with poor posture may be susceptible to frequent injuries or may not perform to the best of his or her ability due to the restrictions that poor posture may present.

Poor posture is usually caused by disease, bad postural habits or is a hereditary condition. A sports massage therapist will only be able to help with poor posture that has come about because of a bad habit, for example, that of slumping forward when sitting at a desk. In this instance, if the action is constantly repeated, then the muscles involved will become accustomed to this position and it may be difficult or painful to return to a normal posture. Poor posture will lead to the muscles being out of balance and will result in fatigue and unnecessary strains being placed upon the body.

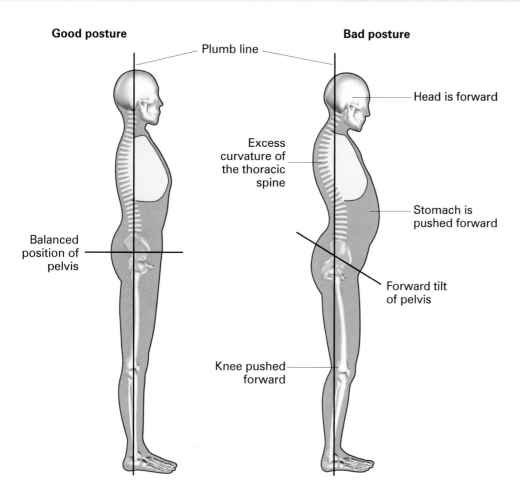

Figure 3.10 *Good and poor posture*

Standing posture is maintained by the antigravity muscles, which give the body its upright position. These are the hamstrings, gluteals, gastrocnemius, erector spinae, illiopsoas, pectorals, rectus femoris, rectus abdominis, quadriceps, longus coli and the trapezius.

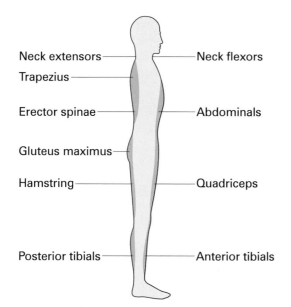

Figure 3.11 *Muscles of postural alignment*

Postural problems caused by bad postural habits can be corrected by exercises that strengthen the specific muscles involved.

During your client consultation, you should note the way in which your client walks and carries him- or herself, along with the way in which he or she sits. A quick postural analysis can be carried out to identify any postural deviations. This can be undertaken in either of two ways: the first involves assessing your client while he or she is lying on the couch and the second involves using a plumb line to represent the line of gravity and assessing the body in the upright standing position.

Assessment of posture with your client on the couch

With your client lying face down and arms at the sides, assess the condition of the spine from the head of the couch and then from the bottom of the couch. Check the position of the pelvis and the position of the knees. Assess your client from the side if necessary. Turn your client over and check body alignment.

Assessment of posture using a plumb line

1 Make your client feel at ease and explain that you are going to conduct a basic postural analysis to identify any postural problems so that exercises can be tailored to his or her needs to help correct the problem and prevent the condition from worsening.

2 Ask your client to undress (preferably behind a curtain or screen), leaving his or her undergarments on.

3 Ask your client to stand facing the wall and ensure that the plumb line passes down the middle of your client's back to assess the rear view.

4 Ask your client to remain still and stand at least ten feet behind the plumb line. Observe and assess your client's posture.

5 After you have assessed the posterior view, ask your client to make a quarter turn to the left and then to the right to analyse posture from the side. In this position, the plumb line must pass through the centre of the shoulder and hip to the anklebone.

A postural fault is noted when a body part considerably deviates in front, behind or away from the plumb line. There are many postural deviations that can be detected using a basic plumb line, which represents the vertical gravity line. The following can be detected when the assessment of your client is undertaken from the lateral view.

Head thrust

This is a common postural fault which results in the head poking forward of the vertical gravity line.

Causes of head thrust

Head thrust is caused through bad postural habits and can be acquired through:

□ slouching

□ watching TV with the head forward

□ driving with the head extended forward

□ straining to listen with the neck extended.

! CONSULTATION FACT

Posture can also be assessed while the client is seated. In this instance, you need to walk around the client, assessing from the front, back and sides. In any postural analysis, consider the position of:

□ head   □ spine

□ neck   □ hips

□ shoulders   □ hands

□ scapula   □ knees

□ clavicle   □ feet

▶ ACTION POINT: HEAD THRUST

Working in pairs as the therapist and the client, encourage the client to think tall and practise holding the head in the correct position. Give after-care advice to the client, which may include home exercises.

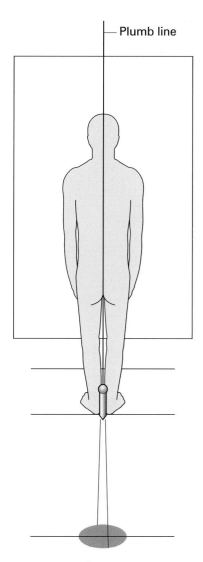

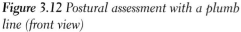

Figure 3.12 *Postural assessment with a plumb line (front view)*

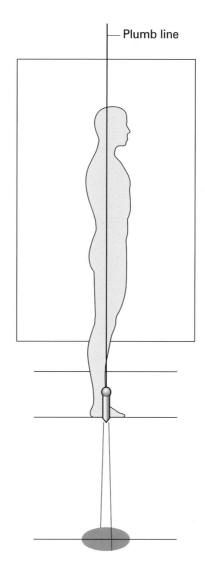

Figure 3.13 *Postural assessment with a plumb line (side view)*

Kyphosis

Kyphosis is an outward curvature of the thoracic spine. With this condition, round shoulders are usually present, that is, the shoulders are rolled forward. There are two types of kyphosis: Type 1 and Type 2.

Type 1

Characteristics include:

- distinctive head thrust
- sagging shoulders
- round shoulders
- slight outward curvature of the thoracic spine
- slight lordosis may be present.

Type 2

Characteristics include:

- head thrust
- a marked lumbar lordosis
- protruding stomach
- prominent round back
- tips of the shoulders sag forward.

Causes of kyphosis

- ☐ Slumping forward when sitting at a desk or using a computer.
- ☐ Straining to see or hear, which results in slumping forward.
- ☐ During puberty when the breasts are developing, some girls may feel self-conscious and adopt a position to hide the breasts, usually a forward position with the shoulders rolled in front of their body.
- ☐ Lack of activity or exercise.

▶ **ACTION POINT: KYPHOSIS**

With guidance from your tutor, demonstrate passive, active, assisted or resisted exercises to:

- ☐ stretch the pectoral muscles
- ☐ strengthen the upper back and neck
- ☐ strengthen the rectus abdominis
- ☐ retract the shoulders.

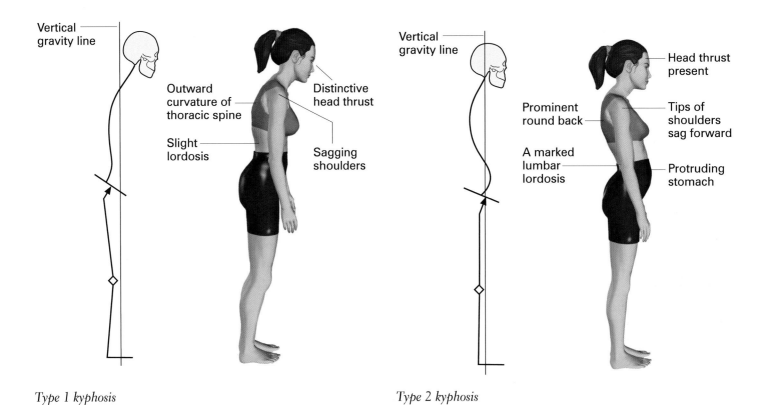

Type 1 kyphosis   *Type 2 kyphosis*

Figure 3.14 *Kyphosis*

Lumbar Lordosis

Lordosis is an inward curvature of the lumbar spine. Lumbar lordosis puts a strain on the back because the bottom is pushed out and the lower back curves inward.

Causes of lumbar lordosis

☐ Being overweight

☐ Pregnancy

☐ Sleeping on the stomach on a soft bed will result in the front of the body, especially the stomach, being pressed into the bed with the bottom sticking out.

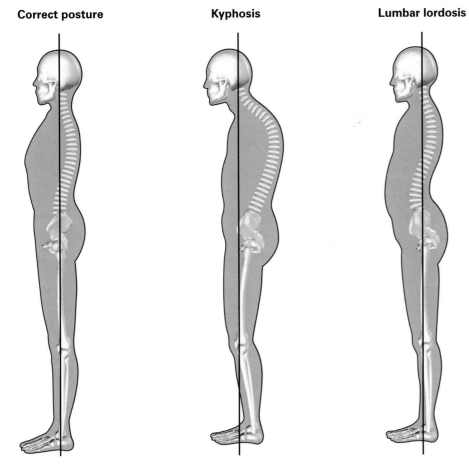

| Correct posture | Kyphosis | Lumbar lordosis |

Figure 3.15 Lumbar lordosis

▶ **ACTION POINT: LUMBAR LORDOSIS**

With guidance from your tutor, demonstrate passive, active, assisted or resisted exercises to:

☐ encourage pelvic tilt

☐ strengthen the abdominals

☐ stretch the back

☐ stretch the hamstrings and hip flexors.

Scoliosis

This postural deviation can be observed from both the front and rear view, with the plumb line representing the vertical gravity line and passing through the middle of the back to the ground. If there are postural problems present, they will deviate from the plumb line and are called lateral faults.

Scoliosis is defined as a lateral curvature of the spine. As well as by using a plumb line, it can be identified by the following method.

1 Identify the prominent structures of the vertebrae of the spine by touch.

2 Place a series of dots using a washable crayon or eyeliner in the centre of each vertebrae from the thoracic vertebrae T1 to the lumbar vertebrae L5.

3 Place a dot on each side of the sacral curve (as illustrated in figure 3.16).

4 Ask your client to lean forward, head dropped, and with hands reaching towards the toes. Observe their action.

5 With the client in an upright position, ask him or her to lean to the left and then to the right, all the time looking for structural changes. If the dots move considerably away from the spine, then scoliosis may be present.

6 Mild scoliosis may be identified when your client bends forward and one shoulder is held higher than the other.

7 Note and record your observations.

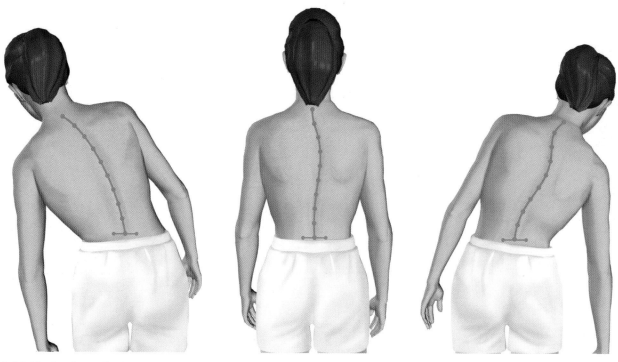

Figure 3.16 Testing for scoliosis

Causes of scoliosis

▢ Carrying a baby on the hip, which causes the posture to be altered.

▢ Carrying a heavy bag repeatedly on one side.

▢ Using one side of the body for specific sports.

▢ Differences in leg length.

To test the flexibility of the upper lateral muscles to ascertain whether scoliosis affects range of movement and to what degree:

▢ ask your client to stand upright with arms loose at his or her sides

▢ ask your client to slide the right hand down the right side of the body to the knee, whilst keeping the hips still and square to the front

▢ measure the distance between your client's fingertips and knee or ankle and repeat on the other side. Note the differences between the two sides of the body (see figure 3.18).

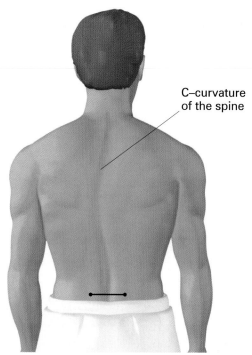

C–curvature of the spine

Figure 3.17 Postural scoliosis

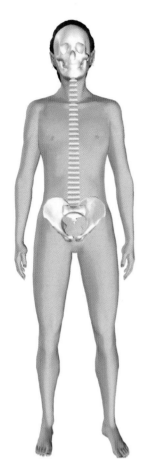
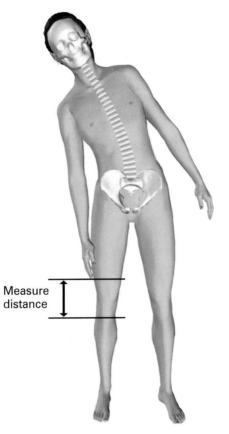

Measure distance

Figure **3.18** *Testing the flexibility of the upper lateral muscles to ascertain whether scoliosis affects range of movement*

> ▶ **ACTION POINT: SCOLIOSIS**
>
> With guidance from your tutor, demonstrate passive, active, assisted or resisted exercises to strengthen and lengthen the spinal muscles.

Flat feet

Flat feet occur where there is a depression of the long arch of the foot. There is usually a gap present on the inner side of the foot when standing. This is the longitudinal arch. If flat feet are present, then there will be a considerably low arch or no arch at all.

Figure **3.19** *Normal and abnormal arches of the foot*

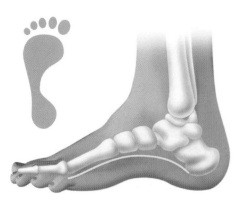

High arch

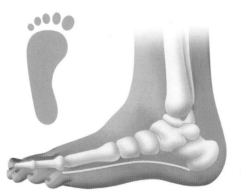

Normal arch

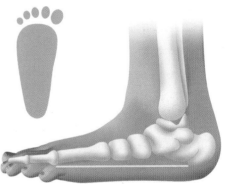

Flat arch

Causes of flat feet

There are many causes of flat feet, which include:

- congenital (born with)
- hereditary
- walking abnormally
- inappropriate shoes
- rupture of ligaments or tendons in the foot
- tight Achilles tendon.

The underlying cause of flat feet must be determined in order to give the right treatment. Congenital and hereditary flat feet will be out of the scope of treatment for a therapist. Non-congenital flat feet, if caught early enough, can be helped by strengthening the intrinsic foot muscles with some of the exercises given below. These exercises should be performed every day for ten to fifteen minutes. If tight Achilles tendons are causing flat feet, then the source of the problem must be tackled first of all. Regular frictions can help to free a tight tendon. The correct walking technique should also be encouraged.

Figure 3.20 Intrinsic foot-muscle strengthening exercises

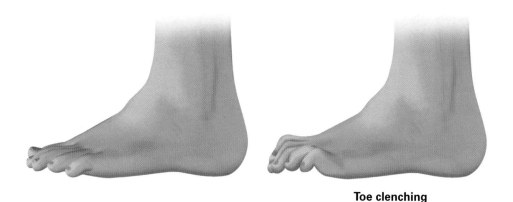

Toe clenching

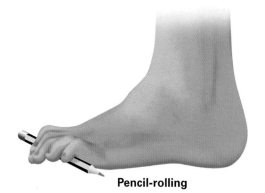

Pencil-rolling

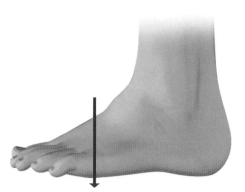

Squeeze toe joints onto floor

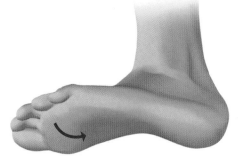

Foot in full inversion, curl toes inwards

▶ ACTION POINT: FLAT FEET

Working in pairs, practise teaching the instrinsic foot strengthening exercises as though you were giving aftercare treatment to a client. Then swap roles.

Flat back

In this condition, no lumbar curve is present. Your client should be asked to try and develop this curve whilst sitting and standing and should also be encouraged to maintain this curve.

Bow-legs

Two variations of bow-legs have been identified: real and apparent. Real bow-legs can be caused by rickets and are outside the scope of a therapist's training. Apparent bow-legs are usually brought about by faulty posture. There will be a medial rotation of the legs and hyperextension of the knees.

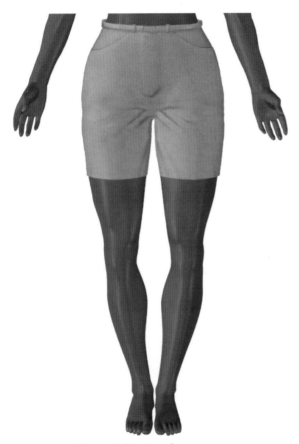

Figure 3.21 Bow-legs

▶ **ACTION POINT:
FLAT BACK**

With guidance from your tutor, demonstrate passive, active, assisted or resisted exercises to:

☐ stretch hamstrings

☐ encourage sitting or standing with a natural postural curve.

▶ **ACTION POINT: BOW-LEGS**

Practise the following exercises for bow-legs with a partner, one working as the therapist and the other as the client.

☐ Place something in between the knees, for example, a newspaper, and ask your client to squeeze.

☐ Ask your client to walk with a football between the legs, which will cause him or her to produce a gripping action.

☐ Work the upper leg to bring the knees in line.

Knock-knees

When your client is standing upright, ask him or her to bring the feet together and allow the medial borders of the knees to touch. If knock-knees are present, then you will notice that the medial borders of the ankle of each foot will not be able to touch each other.

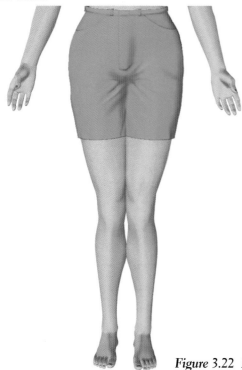

Figure 3.22 *Knock-knees*

Back-knees

This is a hyperextension of the knees; gymnasts usually adopt this position before starting a routine. Back-knees can also be found in people who are obese or overweight.

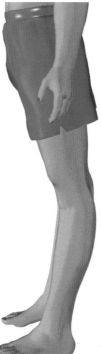

Figure 3.23 *Back-knees*

▶ **ACTION POINT: KNOCK-KNEES**

Practise the following exercises for knock-knees with a partner, one working as the therapist and the other as the client.

☐ A towel or paper should be placed between the ankles and your client then asked to squeeze and strengthen the ankles.

☐ Your client should also be encouraged to walk correctly.

▶ **ACTION POINT: BACK-KNEES**

With guidance from your tutor, develop exercises or activities to:

☐ strengthen the posterior flexors

☐ encourage the correct standing position

☐ encourage bending the knees with feet flat on the floor.

Tibial torsion

This common condition is evident when the knees appear to be winking at each other and is a result of the tendons supporting the knee becoming slack.

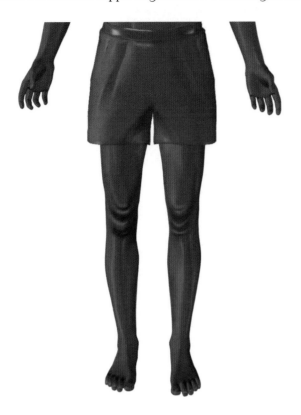

Figure 3.24 Tibial torsion

> ▶ **ACTION POINT: TIBIAL TORSION**
>
> With guidance from your tutor, demonstrate passive, active, assisted or resisted exercises to:
>
> ☐ strengthen the abductors
> ☐ draw the knees back (isometric).

Prominent abdomen

This can be caused by slumping, muscle laxity or an increase in weight.

A sports massage therapist, depending on the extent of the training undertaken, may be able to prescribe strengthening or mobilization exercises to help correct a postural problem that is caused by a bad habit alone. A weight loss programme may also be advised.

> ▶ **ACTION POINT: PROMINENT ABDOMEN**
>
> With guidance from your tutor, demonstrate exercises to:
>
> ☐ mobilize the pelvis
> ☐ take the pressure off the lower back by means of exercises performed in water.

▶ **KNOWLEDGE CHECK**

1 What is a code of ethics? Give four reasons why they are put in place by governing bodies.

2 List five dos and don'ts of personal presentation and state how your appearance affects the 'image' of the workplace.

4 Describe the Health and Safety at Work Act 1974 and state what relevance it has within the working environment of a sports therapist.

5 Describe two other Acts or Regulations that may affect the day-to-day running of a clinic.

6 Describe each element of a client consultation.

7 What can cause postural problems?

8 Describe lumbar lordosis and list the possible causes.

9 How would you recognize a client with kyphosis?

10 List three bad habits that can cause kyphosis.

Preparing the
environment

As a sports massage therapist, you will work in many different environments, including crowded changing rooms, providing massage before and after a game, event or competition. This might mean working on the sidelines of a rugby or football pitch with limited equipment. Wherever you are working, you must always maintain your professionalism and health, safety and hygiene standards.

Since you may not always be able to provide treatment in the comfortable surroundings of the clinic, it is important to build up a quick rapport with your client in order for him or her to feel comfortable with you wherever you are working. Wherever you are treating clients, the necessary materials, such as lubricants, must be to hand.

The clinic environment

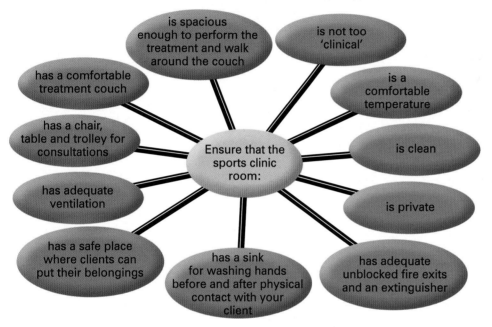

Figure 4.1 Essential properties of a treatment room

When working in a clinic environment you will almost definitely be working in a treatment room specifically designed for therapies. You must ensure that:

The room is not too 'clinical'

The treatment room should be welcoming and not look too much like a hospital.

The room is at a comfortable temperature

Your client may have to undress, so ensure that the room is at a comfortable temperature, not too cold and not too hot.

The room is clean

The therapy room and equipment must be cleaned on a regular basis. Oil spillages should be wiped up as soon as possible in order to prevent accidents occurring.

The room is private

The room should be private and free from people wandering through. Ensure that there is a notice on the door which states that treatment is in progress.

The room is spacious enough to perform the treatment and walk around the couch

The room must be of a good size and large enough to contain the couch, trolley, table and chairs (if possible) – as well as your client and yourself! You need to ensure that you are able to walk around the couch to perform the massage effectively.

In addition, a treatment room should have:

A comfortable treatment couch

The treatment couch must be comfortable for your clients, long enough for a variety of heights and wide enough for a variety of body types. The couch must be in good working order, secure, squeak-free and, if possible, have a face or breathing hole. It is also important to have a couch with an adjustable backrest because some clients may not feel comfortable lying flat.

A chair, table and trolley for consultations

If possible, the treatment room, depending on the size, must have a table and two chairs. Your client will need to feel comfortable and relaxed during the consultation process. Try not to sit behind the table, which would present a rather formal image, but sit next to and slightly facing your client. There should also be a trolley containing everything you need to perform a successful and effective treatment. It is important to move the trolley around with you whilst treating a client; otherwise, you will have to keep leaving your client in order to fetch the oils or creams you need.

Adequate ventilation

The room must be well ventilated but not too breezy. Air conditioning can be turned on low or windows opened slightly.

A safe place where clients can place their belongings

Clients may have to take off their jewellery for some forms of treatment. A good idea would be to place an empty bowl on your trolley for this purpose.

Adequate unblocked fire exits and an extinguisher

Fire exits must be visible and accessible and not blocked by equipment.

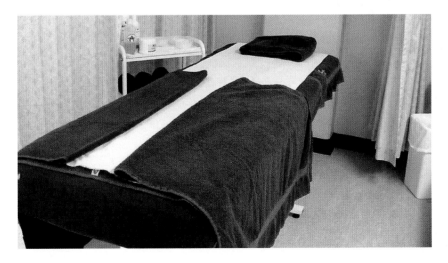

Ensure that the treatment room is comfortable and welcoming

Products required in a clinic environment to successfully perform a treatment

You should ensure that you have the following products and equipment to hand before carrying out a massage treatment.

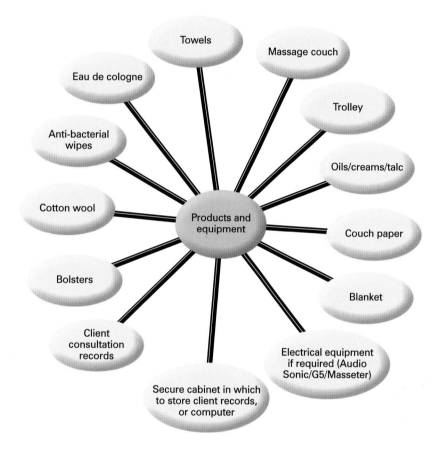

Figure 4.2 *Products required in a clinic environment*

Special note: oils

Increasingly, more and more people now suffer from allergies. It is important to ask your client during consultation whether he or she suffers from any allergies or is allergic to the cream or oils that you are intending to use. The oil is absorbed by the skin and could produce adverse reactions. Almond oil is one of the most popular types of oil; however, it could be life-threatening to someone who has severe allergic or anaphylactic reactions to almonds or other nuts. Oils that could be used instead of almond oil are grapeseed, soya, or a pure vegetable oil.

At the end of the treatment always ask if your client would like the oil or cream to be removed. This can be done by either using cologne or by using a wet but warm towel to wipe off any excess oil. Talcum powder may be used in some instances when your client does not want oil; for instance, when performing inter-event massage during a gymnastics competition, it would not be appropriate to apply oil to a gymnast in between events due to its slippery nature.

Preparing for treatment

Couch

Always ensure that the couch is prepared for treatment prior to your client arriving. It is important to preserve the life of your couch by using adequate covering. A couch cover is inexpensive and will prevent lubricants dripping on to the couch.

> **❗ HEALTH AND SAFETY FACT**
>
> Ensure that the couch is at a suitable height for you. Having a couch that is too low or too high will not allow you to perform the treatment correctly and will also result in undue stresses being placed upon your body, specifically your back.

Couch preparation

- ☐ Couch cover
- ☐ One or two large towels
- ☐ Couch paper
- ☐ Towels for the areas not being treated.

Trolley preparation

- ☐ Couch paper lining the shelves of the trolley
- ☐ Lubricant (oils/creams, spatula)
- ☐ Bowl with wet cotton wool
- ☐ Bowl with dry cotton wool
- ☐ Bowl for client's jewellery
- ☐ Eau de cologne/spirit
- ☐ Anti-bacterial wipes (for the feet)
- ☐ Four bolsters.

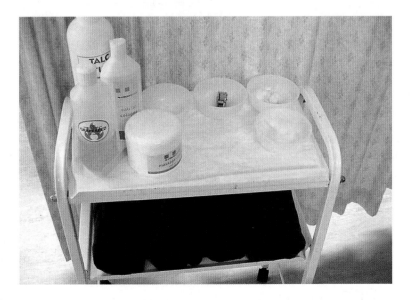

A well-stocked trolley should be kept clean and tidy

Preparing your client for massage

Following the initial consultation, you should:

☐ guide your client to the changing area and ask him or her to remove his or her clothes. Depending upon the area being treated, it may not be necessary to remove all of the clothes; instruct your client accordingly

☐ inform your client how you would like him or her to be positioned on the couch. Give him or her a towel to cover him- or herself in order to maintain his or her modesty

☐ arrange or rearrange towelling to ensure that your client's modesty is maintained and to keep him or her warm.

The initial effleurage or exploratory palpations will enable you to feel the tissues and decide upon the course of treatment.

Preparing to massage the front of the leg

This photograph shows the preparation of a client when performing a leg massage; bolsters are used to support the ankle and knee joints.

Preparing to massage the back of the leg

Bolsters are used for support at the ankle. Towels cover all other areas not being treated.

Preparing to massage the abdomen

For a female client, the towels are positioned to cover the breasts and the hips. For a male client, the towels cover the lower half of the body from the hips down.

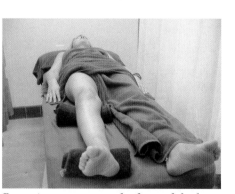
Preparing to massage the front of the leg

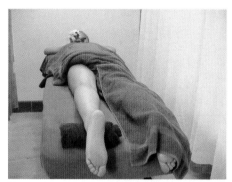
Preparing to massage the back of the leg

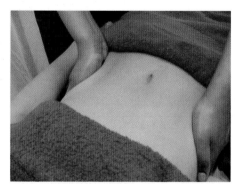
Preparing to massage the abdomen

Preparing to massage the buttocks

Position the towels in order to maintain your client's modesty. Massaging the buttocks can also be performed when massaging the back of the legs; in this instance, the whole leg and buttock would be revealed.

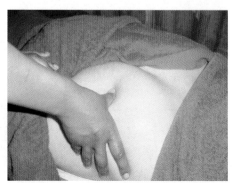
Preparing to massage the buttocks

Preparing to massage the chest

For a female client, the towels are positioned to cover the breasts. For male clients, the towels are positioned to cover the abdomen.

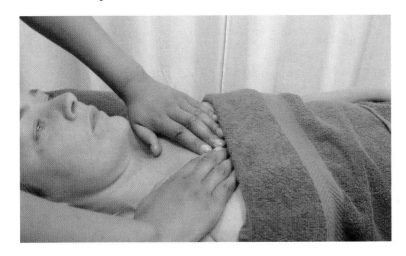

Preparing to massage the chest

Preparing to massage the back

The towels are positioned to expose the whole of the back.

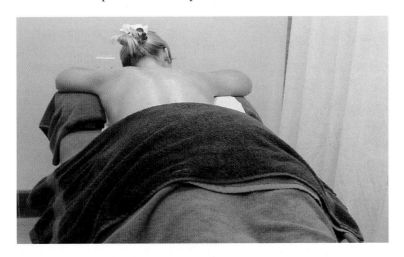

Preparing to massage the back

Preparing to massage the arm

Your client's upper chest and arm are exposed.

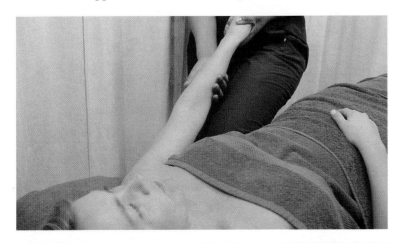

Preparing to massage the arm

Performing massage in a changing-room environment

As a therapist you may be required to work in a changing-room environment. This may be before a game when players are getting ready or it may be at half-time when players are having a pep talk from their coach. In both of these instances, the changing room may be crowded with people so it will be important for you not to get in the way of players but to act professionally and to complete the task in hand.

In a crowded changing room, you may have to kneel on the floor and rest the athlete's leg on your thigh and perform the massage in this position. Make use of your environment – if there is a chair, use it to perform a seated massage if necessary. You will need to be able to adapt your massage quickly to any given situation.

There will not be time to sit down and do a full client consultation; however, you must find out if your client has any major contraindications to treatment and remember that you will or may treat what would be contraindications to other forms of treatment. Ask questions and retain the answers as these can be written up later. Do not forget that in this environment you will be working quickly, but you should also know and have massaged the athletes before.

> ❗ **MASSAGE FACT**
>
> Never massage an athlete for the first time before or during an event. Athletes are all different from each other and their bodies and muscles will react differently to treatment.

The initial effleurage will enable you to feel the area and decide on the techniques to use.

If there is a bench in the changing room, use it. Sit the athlete down or get him or her to lie down, depending on the area being treated. Use towels to cover the bench if necessary.

In an allocated part of a changing room there may be an area with a couch designated for treatments. Use it as if working in a clinic environment.

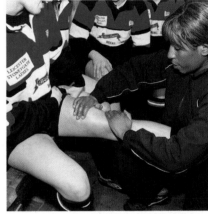

Massaging the quadriceps in a crowded changing room

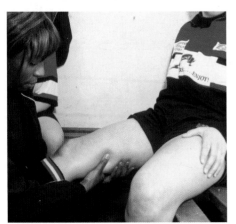

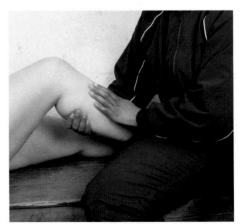

The therapist may have to improvise in a crowded changing room

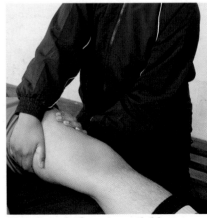

Use a couch if one is available

Performing massage on the field

Some massage may be performed on the pitch at half-time. Use towels for the athletes to sit or lie on. There will not be anywhere to wash your hands, so it is important to carry a bag with you that contains anti-bacterial wipes for your hands to be used after contact with a player. Hygiene standards must always be maintained. The bag must also contain the tools that you may need, such as strapping and lubricants (see page 102 for contents).

If you are the therapist and first-aider for a local football or rugby team, it is important that you stay in the dug-out or behind the sidelines and do not run on the pitch straight away when a player falls or is injured. You must wait for a signal from the referee. It is important to stay alert and watch the game. It is also important to watch the game to observe how the players are performing; watching may allow you to see exactly how a specific injury has occurred.

> **! MASSAGE FACT**
>
> It is essential that you obtain feedback from the client about the treatment that they are being given. Further physical examinations to ascertain the effectiveness of the treatment should also be carried out

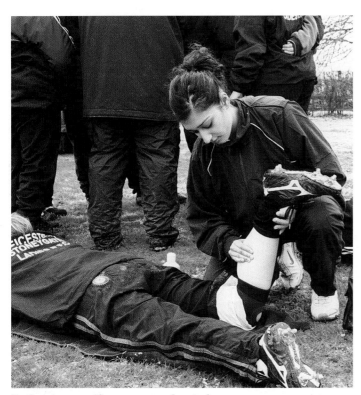

Performing a calf massage on the pitch

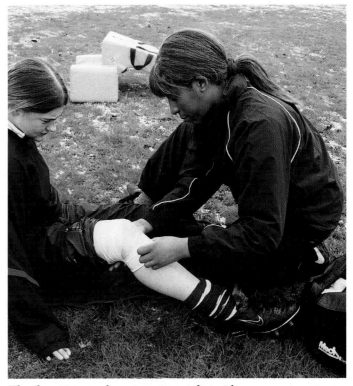

The therapist may have to carry out first aid

Contents of a sports massage bag (including first-aid equipment)

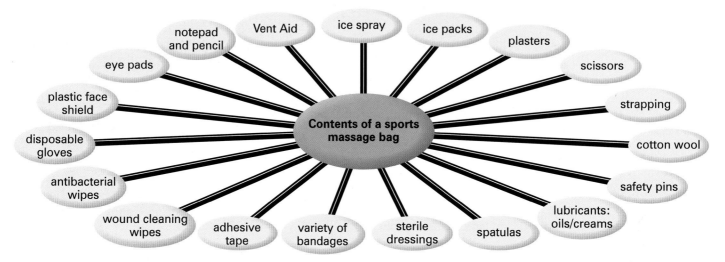

Figure 4.3 Essential contents of a sports massage bag

▶ KNOWLEDGE CHECK

1 Why is it important to maintain health, safety and hygiene standards in all of the different working environments?

2 Why is it important to maintain a professional attitude at all times?

3 Compare and contrast the differences when providing sports massage on the field, in the changing room, and in a dedicated treatment room.

4 List the products that you would need to be able to perform a successful treatment in a clinic environment.

5 Why is it important to have a treatment couch at the right height?

6 List six items that can be found in a sports massage bag.

7 Why might almond oil be life-threatening to some clients?

8 How is a trolley prepared for treatment?

9 After consultation, what are the steps involved in preparing the client for treatment in the clinic environment?

10 Discuss how you might work in a crowded changing room.

▶ ACTION POINT

1 Practise setting up a trolley and a couch ready for treatment.

2 Practise massaging using a chair and a bench. Identify the best position for you to be in when massaging the following:

☐ hamstrings (back of the thigh)

☐ quadriceps (front of the thigh)

☐ back

☐ neck.

NB Always ensure that your client is comfortable and well supported.

- Effleurage

- Petrissage

- Tapotement

- Rocking

- Shaking

- Direct pressure

Classification of massage
techniques

In sports massage, movements are classified into different types.

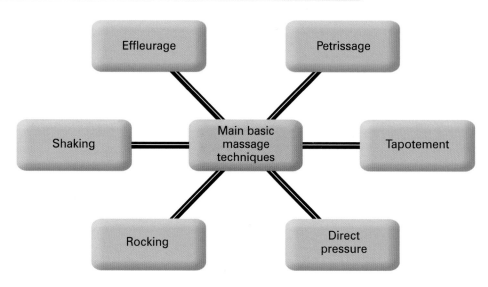

Figure 5.1 *The main basic massage techniques*

The photographs in this section illustrate the different massage techniques. Arrows indicate how the therapist's hands should move during the massage.

➡️   shows the direction of the hands as they move over the body.

▪▪➡️   shows the direction of the hands when they lift off the body.

Remember that these photographs can only indicate how a sports massage should be performed – they are no substitute for watching or performing the real thing!

Effleurage

This is usually the first movement performed in massage. It is used to quickly warm the muscle tissue and spread the lubricant being used. An effleurage is performed using the palmar surface of the hand and the initial strokes will allow the therapist to feel for any trauma that may be present in the muscle tissue. An effleurage can be superficial or deep.

> **❗ MASSAGE FACT**
>
> With all massage techniques, pressure should always be applied towards the heart and reduced on the return stroke.

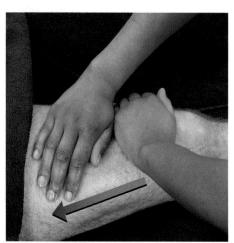

Effleurage of the front quadriceps

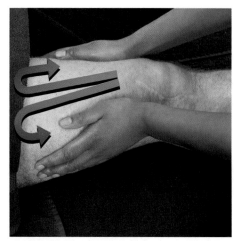

Return phase

Superficial effleurage

Superficial effleurage is a light stroking movement. The therapist allows the hands to slowly stroke and mould the contours of the body part being massaged. The effleurage should be performed with an evenly maintained and light pressure, which usually induces relaxation. Upward sweeping movements are performed in the direction of the lymph nodes, which promotes lymphatic drainage, and the pressure may be slightly increased at the end of the movement to encourage this.

Benefits of superficial effleurage

- Psychologically relaxing.
- Blood and lymph flow locally increased.
- Stimulates lymphatic drainage.
- Stimulates nerve endings.
- Improves blood circulation.
- Used to link other techniques.

Deep effleurage

Deep effleurage is similar to superficial effleurage, the only difference being the depth of pressure that is used and some of the benefits it provides. During sports massage on the pitch, a moderate to deep effleurage is often used, where in a pre-event situation it would be performed quickly to produce a stimulating effect on the muscle tissues. A superficial effleurage is more likely to be used in a therapeutic body massage routine. The speed as well as the pressure applied will alter depending on the objectives of treatment – pre- or post-event massage.

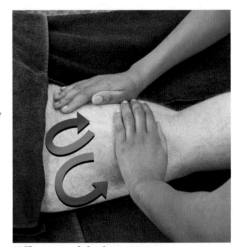

Effleurage of the hamstrings

Benefits of deep effleurage

- Improves blood circulation.
- Improves lymphatic circulation.
- Relaxes contracted muscles.
- Aids the removal of waste products from muscle tissue.
- Aids venous return.

When to use effleurage in sports massage

- In pre-, inter- and post-event massage.
- As the first stroke performed.
- To spread the lubricant being used.
- To introduce your client to touch.
- To put your client at ease.
- To link other techniques.
- As a palpatory method – allows you to feel and sense any tissue abnormalities.

Stroking

Stroking is a technique that is grouped with effleurage and, as its name suggests, it involves stroking the parts of the body being treated. Like effleurage, stroking can be superficial or deep and it can be performed using various parts of the hands and arm. Stroking can be performed in any direction along a muscle, following the direction of the muscle fibres, or transversally – across the length of the fibres. After one stroke, the hands are lifted away from the client's body and returned to the start position to begin the technique again.

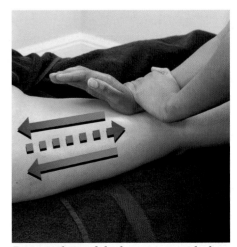

Deep stroking of the hamstrings with the heel of the hand

Stroking using the palmar surface of the hand

This technique using the palmar surface of the hand is very similar to the basic effleurage technique. It can be applied along the longitudinal length of a muscle or it can be applied against the direction of the muscle fibres transversally. This technique can be applied superficially or deeply, to alter the pressure; the stroke is reinforced by placing the other hand, palm down, on the hand that is treating the area.

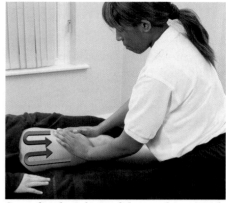

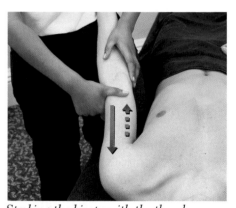

Superficial stroking of the quadriceps with the palms of the hand

Pads of the fingers and pad of thumb

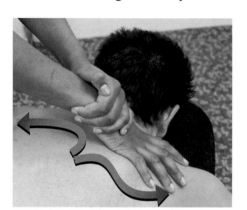

Stroking of the trapezius using fingers and palm

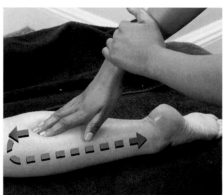

Digital stroking of the calf

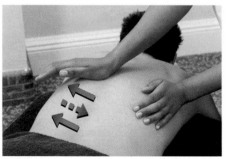

Stroking the biceps with the thumbs

Stroking can be applied using the pads of one, two, three or four fingers. Using one finger, stroking can be applied to smaller muscular areas. Using the pads of the fingers or thumb can provide a deep stroking action. Again, this method will allow the therapist to feel and identify any trauma in the muscle tissue.

Heel of the hand

With the fingers pointing upwards, the heels of the hands can be used to apply a deep stroke to muscle tissue. To reinforce or make the stroke deeper, clasp the hands palm down and apply pressure through both hands.

Forearm

Due to its length, the forearm can sit across the belly of a muscle while applying strokes longitudinally. The therapist's body weight and adjusting the position of the forearm will allow the depth of pressure to be altered.

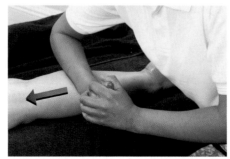

Deep transverse stroking with the heel of the hand

Stroking the calf with the forearm

Elbow

Because of its bony prominence, the elbow is ideal for performing deep stroking. It can be used in areas of tension or where deep work is required. By using slow strokes on areas such as the erector spinae, the muscle that runs parallel to the spine, the therapist will be able to feel for any knots or adhesions that may be present.

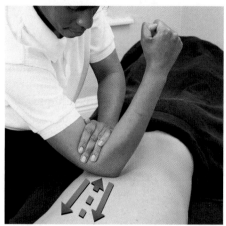

Deep stroking of the erector spinae with the elbow

Ulnar border of a clenched fist

Again, this technique can be used to apply superficial or deep strokes to larger areas of muscle tissue.

Benefits of superficial stroking

- ☐ Psychologically relaxing.
- ☐ Produces a sedative effect.
- ☐ Blood and lymph flow locally increased.
- ☐ Stimulates lymphatic drainage.
- ☐ Stimulates nerve endings.
- ☐ Improves blood circulation.
- ☐ May relieve pain.

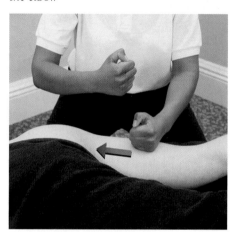

Ulnar border of a clenched fist

Benefits of deep stroking

- ☐ The therapist can assess muscle tissue and identify areas of trauma.
- ☐ Vasodilation of capillaries, which in turn increases the circulation to the area being massaged.
- ☐ Stimulates nerve endings.
- ☐ Loosens muscle tissue.
- ☐ Can stretch the tissue.
- ☐ Can provide a deep penetrative treatment.
- ☐ Can break down adhesions in muscle tissue.

When to use stroking in sports massage

- ☐ In post-event massage.
- ☐ When superficial or deep pressure is required.
- ☐ When smaller muscular areas need massage, the pads of the fingers or thumb can be used.
- ☐ When deep tissue work is required, the elbow can be used effectively.

Petrissage

There are many different strokes within this category and they usually take the form of kneading-type movements or movements that involve lifting, pressing and releasing muscle tissue with intermittent pressure. Petrissage movements are stimulating and can be performed with both hands or one hand. The pressure used when performing petrissage will vary according to the purpose of the massage and the bulk of the tissues.

Types of petrissage

- ☐ Kneading
- ☐ Wringing
- ☐ Skin rolling
- ☐ Thumb sliding
- ☐ Knuckling

Kneading

This is usually performed using the palmar surface of the hands but can also be performed using the fingers or thumb. Kneading involves compressing and releasing muscle tissue and some kneading resembles the movement used when kneading dough.

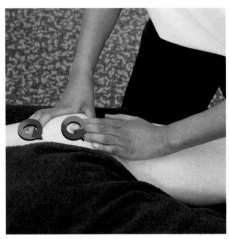

Kneading the gluteals

Palmar kneading

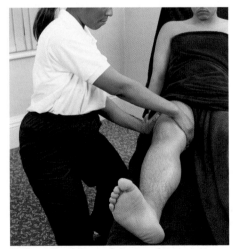

Palmar kneading of the quadriceps

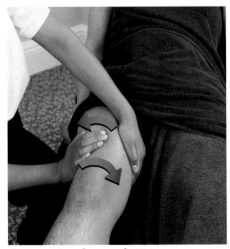

Compressing the muscle tissue

Palmar kneading is usually performed on larger muscle groups such as the hamstrings or quadriceps, where both hands encase the muscle tissue, lifting and compressing sequentially.

Benefits of palmar kneading

- Can be used in pre-event massage to quickly warm major muscle groups.
- Can help relax and loosen muscle tissue.
- Effective in mobilizing muscle tissue.
- Helps to promote lymphatic drainage.
- Can be used in post-event massage.
- Helps to reduce muscle stiffness.
- Stimulates the circulation and increases the blood supply to the muscle.

Thumb or finger kneading/thumb circles

This involves using the pads of the thumb or fingers in a circular motion on the muscle tissue. Using the thumb or fingers can provide a deep pressure massage; again, the pressure must be applied to the upward stroke of the circular movement to promote venous return, and reduced on the downward stroke.

In sports massage, thumb circles are frequently used around the knee joint where it will stimulate the flow of synovial fluid, thereby allowing freer movement.

Thumb or finger kneading can be used on any part of the body and can be used to target specific areas of muscle tissue.

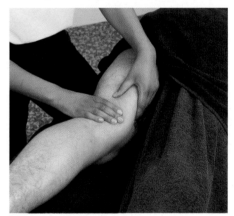

Thumb kneading targets specific areas of the body

Benefits of thumb or finger kneading

- Can be used on small areas where deep pressure is needed.
- Can be used to break down adhesions in muscle tissue.
- Can help to reduce muscle tension in smaller muscular areas.
- Will increase localized circulation of blood and lymphatic drainage.

Reinforced kneading

In reinforced kneading, both hands are used with one on top of the other to increase the depth of the stroke. The kneading in this instance is performed with the heel of the hand. In addition to the uses of kneading previously described, reinforced kneading can give a deep massage to muscular areas or areas where there is a lot of adipose tissue.

Wringing the hamstrings

Wringing

Wringing involves compressing tissue between the thumbs and index fingers of the hands and then lifting and twisting in a figure of eight, passing the tissue alternately from one hand to the other, in quick succession.

Benefits of wringing

- Can be used as part of a pre-event massage where it will be effective in warming and stimulating the muscle tissue quickly.
- Can help to reduce tension and relax muscle tissue when performed as part of a post- event massage.
- Can help to improve and increase localized circulation, which in turn will produce localized heat, which is effective in helping to reduce pain.
- Can stretch muscle fibres and fascia.

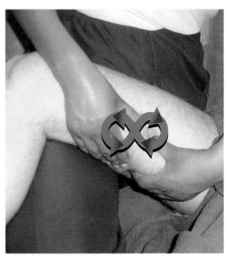

Wringing the adductors

The wringing action can be simulated using one hand with the index finger and thumb being used to lift and compress the tissue. The free hand should be used to support the body part being worked on. This is sometimes known as 'picking up'.

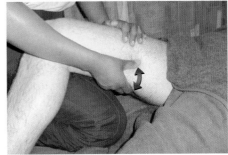

One-handed wringing of the adductors

Skin rolling

Skin rolling, as its name suggests, is rolling of the skin; the fingers and the thumbs are used to lift and roll the skin. This particular skin roll is mainly used in a therapeutic massage treatment where its main function is to move the skin in order to improve its suppleness and pliability. The repeated action results in an increased flow of oxygen-rich blood to the area which, as well as producing an erythema (redness of the skin), will improve the condition of the skin.

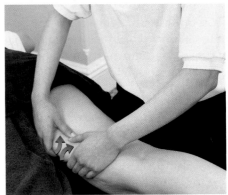

Skin rolling of the hamstrings

Another method of rolling which is more beneficial in a sports massage treatment is muscle rolling. This is where both the skin and muscle is lifted and rolled away from the bone using the radial borders of the hand and thumb. It can be performed using one hand or two.

Benefits of muscle rolling

- ☐ Can help to stretch muscle tissue.
- ☐ Can reduce muscle tension.
- ☐ Increases lymphatic drainage.
- ☐ Increases blood flow to the muscle tissue.
- ☐ Increases the skin's pliability.

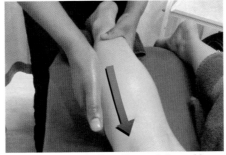

One-handed muscle-rolling of the calf: Step 1

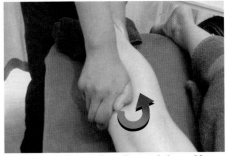

One-handed muscle-rolling of the calf: Step 2

Thumb sliding

This involves sliding the thumb up the length of a muscle. Both thumbs can be used to slide and deeply penetrate the muscle tissue; however, it is important to support the area being treated. If performed using one hand, then in some instances the other can be used to support the limb.

Thumb sliding also has the advantage of being able to stretch muscle tissue, so should not be used on areas where there is excess skin or where there is a great deal of hyper-flexibility (over-pliability). This particular treatment will be beneficial on areas which the athlete or therapist might find difficult to stretch actively or passively.

Benefits of thumb sliding

- ☐ Can be used to stretch muscle tissue.
- ☐ Can help improve muscle elasticity.
- ☐ Can help to disperse lactic acid.
- ☐ Can help to identify muscle adhesion.

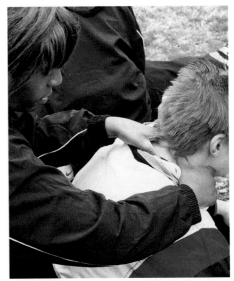

Pitchside thumb sliding of the neck

Knuckling

There are many different methods of knuckling that can be used effectively in sports massage. Knuckling involves using the knuckles of the hand to manipulate muscle tissue.

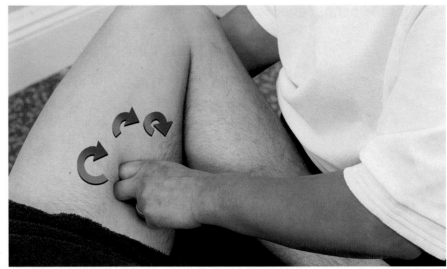

Knuckling the adductors

Knuckle clasp

This involves using the knuckle of the index finger as the primary force, but at the same time, clasping the muscle tissue between the bent knuckle and the thumb and pulling it away from the bone. The movement produced by the knuckle is a circular upward movement, pressure being applied on the upward stroke.

Benefits of knuckle clasp

☐ Can increase local circulation.
☐ Effective in areas where tension nodules are present.
☐ Helps to break down adhesions present in muscle tissue.
☐ Helps to reduce muscle tightness.

Bent knuckling

This technique gives a deep penetration because it is performed with the tip of the knuckle. The knuckle of the index finger alone is used in a circular motion, which allows a more direct pressure to be applied to the muscle.

Benefits of bent knuckling

☐ Deeper treatment.
☐ Direct pressure can be applied.
☐ Effective in reducing tension nodules.
☐ Effective in helping to break down fibrositic nodules found between muscle fibres.

Knuckle twisting

This technique involves using the knuckles of a clenched fist and twisting at the wrist whilst the knuckles strike the muscle tissue.

Benefits of knuckle twisting

☐ Helps to loosen tight muscles.
☐ Reduces muscle tension.
☐ Can give a deep massage.

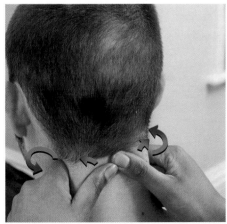

Knuckle roll and thumb clasp of the neck

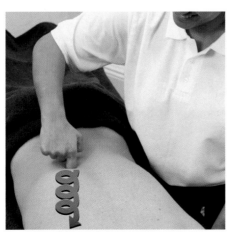

Bent knuckling of the erector spinae

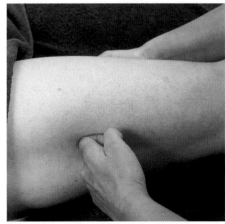

Knuckle twisting of the quadriceps

Heel (of the hand) squeeze

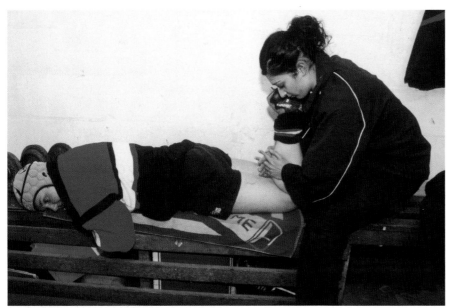

Heel squeeze on the calf in a changing room

The heel squeeze involves compressing or squeezing the muscle between the heels of both hands simultaneously. The heel squeeze can be effectively used on the quadriceps, hamstrings and calf where the belly of the muscle is grasped and compressed.

Benefits of heel squeeze

- Increases the circulation.
- Increases lymphatic drainage.

The squeezing action performed will have different effects on the muscle tissue. When the muscle is squeezed, deoxygenated blood and waste products will be released from the tissue. During the non-compression phase, oxygen-rich blood will flow and deliver nutrients to the muscle tissue.

When to use petrissage in sports massage

- In pre-, inter- and post-event massage.
- When larger muscles need massage.
- When mobilization of muscle tissue is required.
- To stretch muscle fibres and fascia.
- When muscle elasticity needs to be improved.
- When direct pressure is required – knuckling.
- When a deeper manipulation is required on smaller areas, using thumb or finger kneading.
- When loosening of the tissue is needed.

Tapotement

Tapotement is a group of stimulating massage techniques sometimes referred to as percussion because of the rhythmic movement of the hands on the muscle tissue. The tissue is usually struck with both hands alternately. These movements are usually used in a pre-event and inter-event massage when they serve to stimulate the muscle tissue and nerve endings.

Types of tapotement techniques

- Hacking
- Cupping
- Slapping
- Pounding
- Beating

Hacking

This technique is performed using the ulnar border of the hands; both hands should swiftly strike the muscle tissue alternately. Hacking is a stimulating manipulation that is often used in a pre-event situation to stimulate muscle tissue before an activity.

The little, ring and middle fingers are those that strike the tissue. The little finger should be slightly bent inwards as it comes into contact with the tissue. If this technique is performed incorrectly, it can be painful for the client.

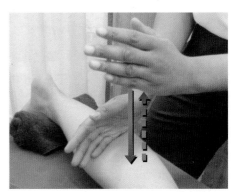
Hacking the calf

Cupping

The hands are cupped to perform this technique; the fingers of the hands are closed and bent at the knuckle to form an arch. The thumbs rest on the index finger, which should produce a slight gap. Keeping this position, the hands should briskly strike the tissue alternately. If a hollow sound is produced, the tissue is being struck correctly; a slapping sound may mean that the hands are too flat. Cupping is more effective on larger muscle groups.

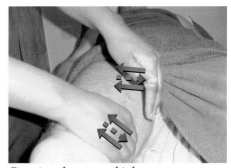
Cupping the upper thigh

Slapping

Slapping is very similar to cupping, but with the hands held flat. The fingers are together and the whole palmar surface of the hand strikes the tissue.

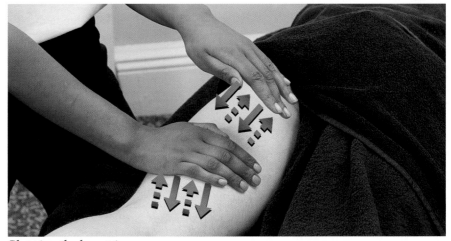
Slapping the hamstrings

Pounding

Whilst rolling the hands over each other, the ulnar borders of clenched fists are used to strike the muscle being treated. Pounding should be used on areas where there is a lot of tissue, for example, the buttocks or hamstrings.

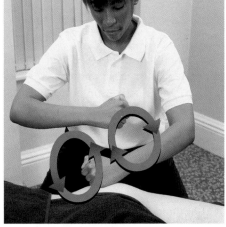

Pounding the gluteals

Beating

This technique is one of the deepest of the muscle strokes and should be used on the large muscle groups of the body. Beating is performed using the ulnar borders of loosely clenched fists. The fists are held in a vertical position and strike the tissue alternately. Beating can also be performed by turning the clenched fist from a vertical to a horizontal position and then striking the muscle tissue with the knuckles.

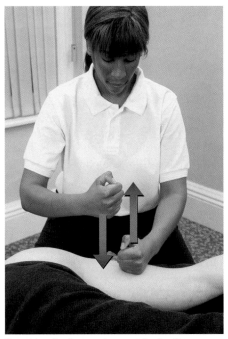

Beating the hamstrings with the fists

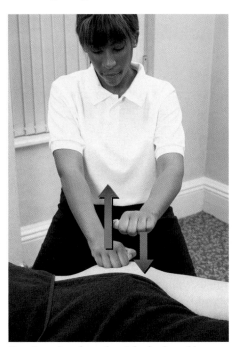

Beating the gluteals with the knuckles

Benefits of tapotement

- ☐ Increased blood flow to the area, due to the repeated action of tapotement, which warms the muscle tissue.
- ☐ Hacking, beating and pounding can produce a deep stimulating effect.
- ☐ Hacking can stimulate nerve endings.
- ☐ Can improve muscle tone.

When to use tapotement in sports massage

- ☐ In a pre-event massage.
- ☐ During an inter-event massage.
- ☐ When a stimulating effect is required.
- ☐ When muscle tone needs to be improved.
- ☐ To relieve muscle spasm.

Rocking

Rocking can be performed using one or both hands, the hands moving back and forth over the muscle tissue. In this technique, the rocking is performed by the heels of both hands applying pressure on the forward motion and the fingertips pulling the tissue on the backward motion. One of the benefits of using rocking in sports massage is that it can quickly relax muscle tissue.

When to use rocking in sports massage

- In post-event massage.
- At the beginning and end of treatment.

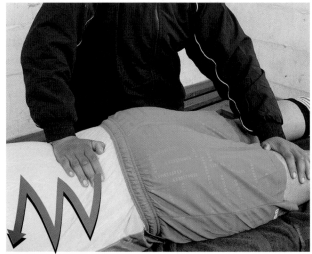

Rocking on the back

Shaking

The muscle tissue is grasped with the palmar surfaces of the hands and shaken from side to side. Shaking will loosen tight muscle tissue and may be used at the end of a post-event massage to quickly relax the muscle tissue. Shaking can also be performed using one hand, with the other used as support for the limb being treated. Using one hand, the fingers or thumb are used to perform the techniques.

Benefits of shaking

- Relaxes muscle tissues.
- Reduces muscle stiffness.
- Stimulates circulation.
- Can help to relieve pain.
- Can stimulate nerve endings.

When to use shaking in sports massage

- Pre-event massage, when the technique would be performed quickly for stimulation purposes.
- Inter-event and pre-event massage.
- Performed slowly in post-event massage to relax the muscles.

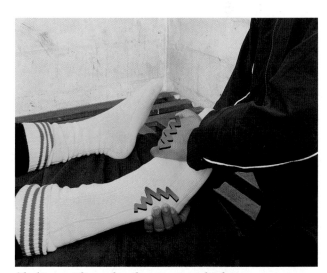

Shaking, with one hand supporting the foot

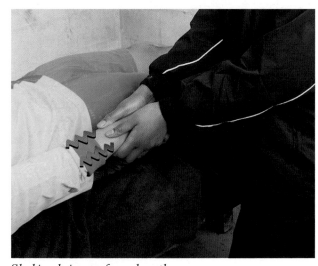

Shaking being performed on the arm

Direct pressure

As its name suggests, direct pressure is a method of applying pressure directly to an area requiring treatment to reduce muscle spasm and relieve areas of tenderness. One of the benefits of direct pressure is that it stimulates the circulation of blood locally. Direct pressure is applied with the pads of the fingers or thumb, or the elbow, and held for between ten and twenty seconds, using a firm, even pressure. As with neuro-muscular techniques, the pressure must be applied gradually. Direct pressure should be followed by passive stretching.

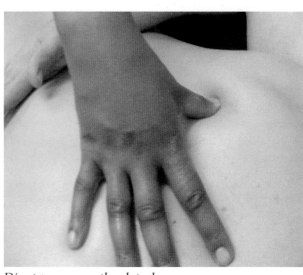

Direct pressure on the gluteals

Benefits of direct pressure

☐ Can help to relieve pain.

☐ Reduces muscle spasm.

☐ Increases local circulation.

When to use direct pressure in sports massage

☐ In post-event massage.

☐ When muscle spasm is present.

☐ When pain relief is necessary.

▶ **KNOWLEDGE CHECK**

1 When should you use effleurage?

2 Give two benefits of superficial effleurage.

3 Give two benefits of deep effleurage.

4 Describe stroking.

5 Compare the differences between stroking using the elbow and stroking using the forearm.

6 Wringing is a technique that is grouped under petrissage. Give four other examples of petrissage.

7 What are the benefits of wringing?

8 What are the benefits of using tapotement in sports massage and when would you use it?

9 Describe four tapotement techniques.

10 How and when would you use shaking?

Performing the

massage

Selecting a massage technique

Unlike a body massage performed as a beauty treatment, there is no specific routine to follow in sports massage. The techniques used in a sports massage depend on personal circumstances, the demands of the sport or activity, and the needs of your client. It is important to discuss the treatment plan with your client prior to the massage. Always allow for opportunities to discuss the appropriateness of the treatment. An effleurage is always used as the initial stroke to warm the tissues and assess the condition of the muscles being treated. As the therapist, you must be able to select and use the techniques that will be the most beneficial for your client. Massage techniques can be quickly adapted to allow you to work through clothes whenever this may be necessary; however, effleurage and some stroking will be difficult.

The following pages detail some of the techniques that can be used during a sports massage. For an easier understanding of how the same technique is performed on different parts of the body, the photographs have been grouped to specifically show the techniques, for example, effleurage, petrissage and tapotement being performed on the legs, arms, chest and back. Some techniques used on the abdomen and neck have also been included. With each photograph, the stance and a description of how to perform the technique is given. For more details on several of the hand positions, see the table opposite.

The following section on event massage (page 137) allows you to see how some of the techniques described are used to massage different clients.

Stance

It is important to adopt the correct stance when massaging your client in order to apply the technique correctly and for your own health and safety. Adopting poor posture could lead to unnecessary strain being placed upon your body; you will become fatigued more quickly if you do not adopt the correct stance.

Massage depth of pressure

Massage depth of pressure

The depth of pressure will vary with each massage performed. It depends on the clients and upon the time when the massage is given (for example, whether it is a pre- or post-event massage).

The depth of pressure can be superficial, moderate, deep, or a mixture of each. With practice, the depth at which to apply a stroke will become natural to you; however, always check with your client that the massage is not unduly painful.

Massage speed and rhythm

A pre-event massage should be performed at a pace that will quickly, but not too quickly, warm up and stimulate the muscle tissues. If a pre-event massage is performed slowly, it may relax your client and could induce sleep, which could be detrimental to his or her performance.

A post-event massage should be performed more slowly than a pre-event massage and should include lots of effleurage, stroking and petrissage techniques. A continuous rhythm should be developed when applying any massage technique.

! MASSAGE FACT

A slow massage will have a calming or sedative effect compared with a quicker massage, which will provide a stimulating effect.

Technique	Hand position	Brief description	Area of body / notes
Transverse palmar kneading		Palms lift and compress the tissues. The hands cross each other.	Can be used on larger muscle groups.
Kneading		Circular movements performed either with fingers or palmar surface of the hands.	Can be used on all areas of the body.
Wringing		Alternately lift and compress the tissue between index finger and thumb in a figure of 8. Use the other fingers to lift and knead the muscle tissue in a circular motion.	Can be performed on the legs, back, neck, buttocks and abdomen. If working on the leg, flex and abduct the client's leg and support it with your body.
One-handed wringing		The muscle tissue is grasped and lifted between index finger and thumb. The remaining fingers move in a kneading and circular motion over the muscle tissue.	As above. If using one-handed wringing on the upper arm, rest the client's arm on your knee.
Skin-rolling		The skin is picked up and rolled away by the thumbs.	Usually performed on the superficial tissues. Deep skin-rolling can also be performed on muscle tissue where a deeper method of application would be used.
One-handed muscle roll		The fingers lift the muscle tissue and the side of the thumb pushes it away. Can also use two hands on either side of the muscle.	Can be performed on the legs, abdomen, muscular areas of the back, biceps and triceps.
Pummelling		The wrist of a tightly clenched fist is moved in a clockwise direction while the flat area of the fist pummels the tissue.	Can be performed on all areas of the body. Pummelling does not involve the use of the knuckles.
Knuckling		The hand and wrist move in a clockwise motion while pressure is applied with the knuckles.	Can be used on all parts of the body. The knuckles should 'run' across the chest, when massaging that area.
Bent knuckling		The bent knuckle of the index finger applies moderate-to-deep pressure. The knuckle is moved in a small circular motion.	A bent knuckle is very effective on areas where tightness is felt.

Table of hand techniques

Heel stroking		The heel of the hand is used to stroke the muscle tissue. Reinforce the stroke by placing one hand on top of the other, interlocking the fingers and pulling the fingers of the top hand back.	Can be used on the larger muscle groups.
Digital stroking		The pads or whole surface of the fingers can be used.	1, 2, 3 or 4 fingers can be used, depending on the size of the area being worked upon.
Palm stroking		The palmar surfaces of the hands stroke the muscle.	
Elbow stroking		The elbow is used as a deep massage technique.	Effective along the erector spinae, buttocks and hamstrings.
Two-handed hacking		Palms of both hands, loosely touching each other, strike the muscle tissue.	Used on larger muscle groups.
Hacking		Alternate hands are used to strike the muscle tissue in a continuous rhythm.	Used on larger muscle groups.
Cupping		Cupped hands alternately strike the muscle in a continuous rhythm.	Used on larger muscle groups.
Pounding		The ulnar borders of clenched fists roll over each other to alternately strike the muscle tissue.	Used on larger muscle groups.
Slapping		Palmar surfaces of the hands alternately strike the muscle in a continuous rhythm.	Used on larger muscle groups.
Beating: vertical fists		Fists are clenched in a vertical position, with the ulnar borders striking the muscle.	Used on larger muscle groups.
Beating: horizontal fists		Fists are clenched. The knuckles and distal parts of the fingers strike the muscle tissue.	Used on larger muscle groups.
Heel squeeze		Hands are clasped together. The belly of the muscle is compressed and released with the heels of the hands.	Used on larger muscle groups.

What is a contraindication?

A contraindication may be described as the existence of a medical condition, ailment, or any other reason why massage should not be applied. For example, epilepsy, diabetes, high blood pressure and heart defects are contraindications to some forms of massage therapy. Massage has different effects on the muscles, bones and joints, circulatory system, lungs, skin, and other body systems. Therefore, certain medical conditions may be worsened by massage treatment. It is important in these cases that you obtain guidance and approval from your client's GP for the treatment to be given. However, there are some medical conditions that are not contraindicated to sports massage. For specific contraindications, refer to the end of each unit in Section 2 on anatomy and physiology.

The importance of client consultation in identifying contraindications

During the consultation phase, you must ask your client if he or she suffers from any contraindications. Some clients will not understand the term contraindication, so explain what it means, as well as listing the conditions that are contraindicated to sports massage. Also ask your client if there are any other conditions that you should know about and check if he or she is currently taking any medication.

Seeking permission from your client's GP

If your client tells you that he or she has a specific condition that you have not heard of, do not be afraid to ask him or her to explain it to you. If there is anything that you are unsure about, seek medical advice or approval from your client's GP before starting a programme of treatment. It is vital that you obtain your client's permission before contacting his or her GP. It is good practice to contact the GP by letter. An example of a letter is given opposite.

The Central Academy of Sports Therapies
Mansfield Road, Leicester LE1 2JP
Telephone: 0116 1111111

Dr Henry
Lectstock Health Centre
Harrington Way
Leicester LE1 2ZZ

Dear Dr Henry,

Re: Patient Daniel Brooks, 15 Churchfield Close, Leicester

D.O.B 23 June 1945

During a recent consultation with Daniel, we discussed his history of very high blood pressure, which is contraindicated in massage. I would appreciate it if you could let me know whether you feel that Daniel would be at risk if receiving massage treatment. I have discussed with him the fact that I cannot treat him without your prior approval.

I look forward to your reply at your earliest convenience.

Yours sincerely,

Janice Anderson
Sports massage therapist

The photographs in this section illustrate the different massage techniques. Arrows indicate how the therapist's hands should move during the massage.

➡️ shows the direction of the hands as they move over the body.

▪▪▶ shows the direction of the hands when they lift off the body.

Remember that these photographs can only indicate how a sports massage should be performed – they are no substitute for watching or performing the real thing!

Applying effleurage, petrissage and tapotement techniques to different parts of the body

Starting to effleurage the leg

Stance   Forward lunge stance; front knee bent, back leg straight

Hand position   Start from the toes, using both hands in a horizontal position; start to effleurage

Technique   Apply pressure in an upward sweeping movement from the toes to the quadriceps. Ensure that the pressure is even on the return phase of this technique. Lunge forward and use your body weight to assist in the application of pressure

Return phase   Draw the front leg back as the hands sweep back towards the toes

NB Effleurage can also be performed with hands in a vertical position, that is, with the fingers pointing towards your client.

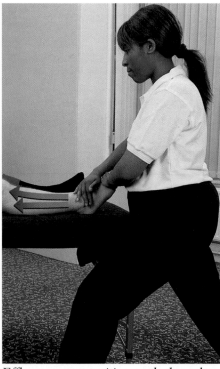

Effleurage: start position on the lower leg

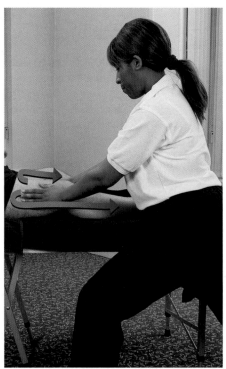

Return phase following the contours of the leg

Effleurage of the quadriceps

Stance	Forward lunge stance
Hand position	Horizontal or vertical to perform the effleurage of the quadriceps
Technique	Apply pressure with an upward stroke, moving the hands over the quadriceps
Return phase	Mould your hands around your client's inner and outer thigh

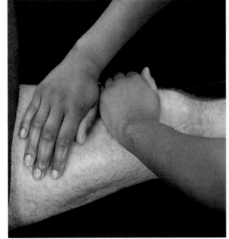 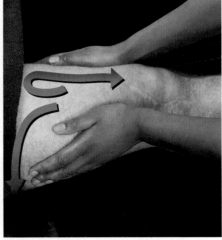

Effleurage of the quadriceps: Step 1   *Effleurage of the quadriceps: Step 2*

Effleurage of the lower leg

Stance	Forward lunge stance
Hand position	Horizontal or vertical to perform the effleurage of the quadriceps
Technique	Apply light pressure in an upward direction, avoiding the knee
Return phase	Follow the contours of the lower leg back to the toes

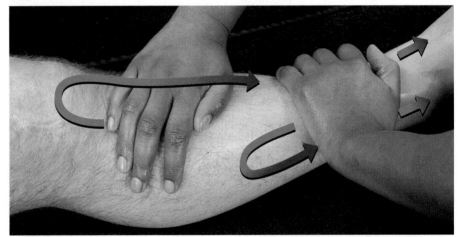

Effleurage of the lower leg

Effleurage of the hamstrings

Stance	Forward lunge stance
Hand position	Horizontal or vertical to perform the effleurage of the quadriceps
Technique	Apply deeper pressure to this muscle group in an upward direction, ensuring that the palms are in contact with the skin at all times
Return phase	Allow the hands to mould against the contours of the upper thigh

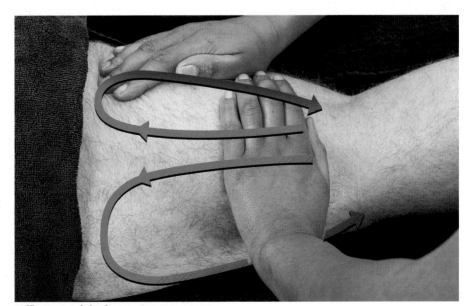

Effleurage of the hamstrings

Effleurage of the arm

Stance   Forward lunge stance

Hand position   Support your client's arm at the wrist

Technique   Start with your hand under the arm at the wrist (supinated position), lifting your client's arm off the couch. Your client's arm is in a pronated position. Cup the arm and sweep in an upward position under the forearm, up and around the triceps

Return phase   Move the hand over the deltoid and bring your hand back over the arm towards the fingertips. Maintain an even pressure. Change your hands to ensure effleurage is performed over the deltoids

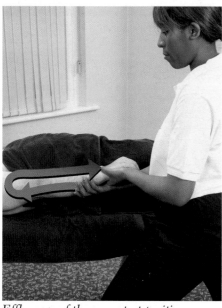

Effleurage of the arm: start position

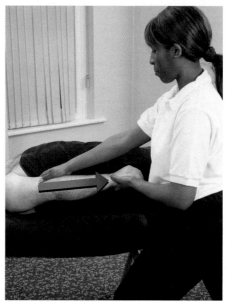

Effleurage of the arm

Alternative effleurage

Stance   Forward lunge stance

Hand position   Horizontal or vertical position. Your client's arm is resting on the couch

Technique   Use the same technique as that identified for the legs

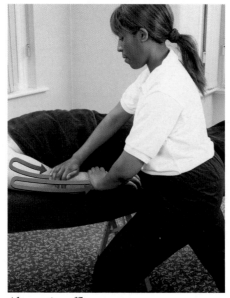

Alternative effleurage

Effleurage of the chest

Stance   Parallel stance at the head of the couch

Hand position Fingertips parallel to the sternum

Technique   Using the whole hand, apply a firm stroke in a 'v' shape up towards the deltoids. Move the hands around the deltoids towards your client's back. The hands stroke the trapezius to the attachment at the occipital bone. Support your client's head in your hands and gently stretch the neck, pulling towards you

NB Do not attempt this technique without supervision or adequate training.

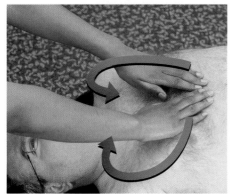
Effleurage of the chest: start position

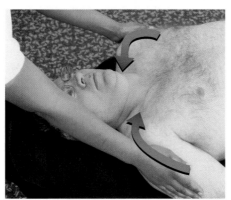
Effleurage of the chest

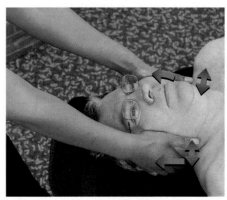
Effleurage of the chest: neck stretch

Effleurage of the neck (seated)

Stance   Stand behind your client

Hand position Clasp the neck in both hands

Technique   Using the whole hand, gently apply a firm upward stroke using the "V" between the thumb and the index finger

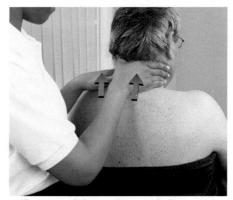
Effleurage of the neck: seated client

Effleurage of the neck (prone)

Stance   Stand adjacent to your client

Hand position Use one hand to support your client's neck and use the index finger and thumb of the other hand

Technique   Apply firm and upward stroking movements to the neck

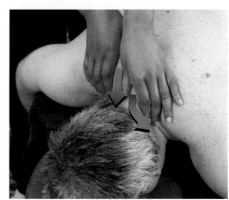
Effleurage of the neck: prone client

Effleurage of the back

Stance	Forward stance, with a slightly bent forward knee
Hand position	Fingertips, starting at the sacrum
Technique	Place your hands flat on your client's back, using an upward stroke along the erectus spinae. Move towards the trapezius and the deltoids
Return phase	Move your hands over the deltoids and the latissimus dorsi back to the sacrum

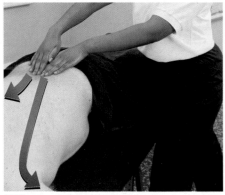 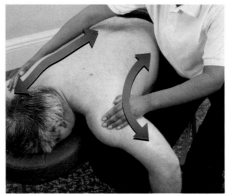 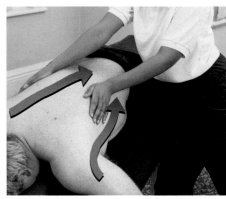

Effleurage of the back: Step 1   *Effleurage of the back: Step 2*   *Effleurage of the back: Step 3*

Transverse palmar kneading of the quadriceps

Stance	Face your client's leg, back straight, tilt pelvis forward and bend knees slightly
Hand position	Refer to table (page 119)
Technique	This is a pick-up-and-push technique. The leg tissue is lifted and compressed between the palms of both your hands. Work up the leg, from the top of the knee region to the top of the thigh

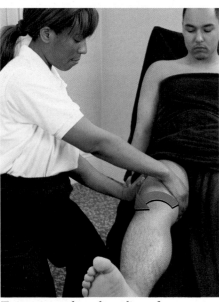 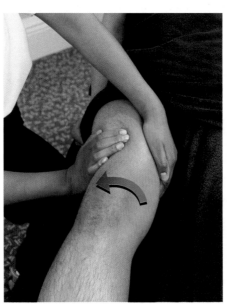

Transverse palmar kneading of the quadriceps   *Transverse palmar kneading of the quadriceps*

Transverse palmar kneading of the calf and hamstrings

Stance   Face your client's leg, back straight, tilt pelvis forward and bend knees slightly

Hand position   Refer to table (page 119)

Technique   Same movement as for the quadriceps

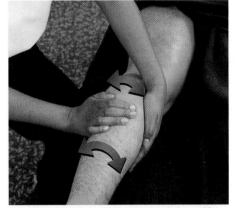

Transverse palmar kneading of the calf

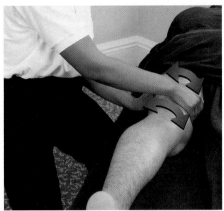

Transverse palmar kneading of the hamstring

Cross-fibre stretch of the back

Stance   Stand facing your client's back

Hand position   Hands either side of the back, fingers facing away from *your* body

Technique   Apply pressure, using the heel of the hand, to compress and stretch the tissue as your hands cross over from one side of the back to the other

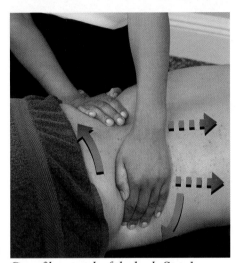

Cross fibre stretch of the back: Step 1

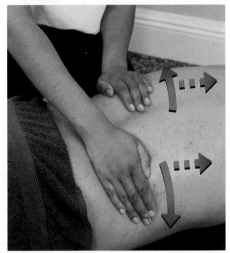

Cross fibre stretch of the back back: Step 2

Wringing of the inner thigh

Stance   Support your client's leg with your body. Kneel on the couch next to your client

Hand position   Refer to table (page 119)

Technique   Grasp the tissue in the palm of your hand, holding it between finger and thumb, lift and move the tissue up and away from the bone in a figure of eight pattern. Move up, down, and across the length of the muscle

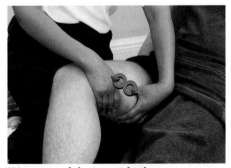

Wringing of the inner thigh

Wringing of the quadriceps

Stance   Stride stance, facing your client's leg

Hand position and technique   Apply the same technique as in wringing of the inner thigh

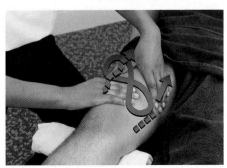

Wringing of the quadriceps

Wringing of the calf and hamstrings

Stance, hand position and technique   Apply the same technique as in wringing of the inner thigh

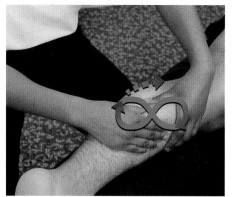

Wringing of the calf

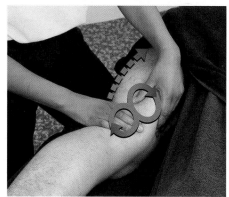

Wringing of the hamstrings

One-handed wringing of the upper arm

Stance	Body adjacent to the couch, with your knee on the couch
Hand position	Refer to table (page 119)
Technique	Rest your client's arm on your knee. Pick up and lift the muscle tissue between the thumb and the index finger and move it in a figure of eight pattern

Wringing of the latissimus dorsi

Stance	Stride stance
Hand position	Refer to table (page 119)
Technique	The technique is the same as in wringing of the quadriceps and calf and hamstrings. Work up the latissimus dorsi, rhomboids, and other deep muscle groups around the scapula

Wringing of the abdomen

Stance	Stride stance
Hand position	Refer to table (page 119)
Technique	Use the same technique as in wringing of other parts of the body.

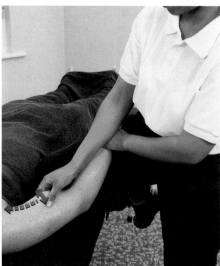

One-handed wringing of the upper arm

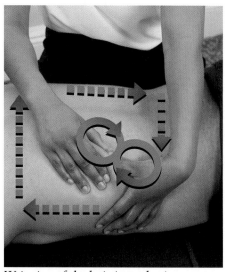

Wringing of the latissimus dorsi

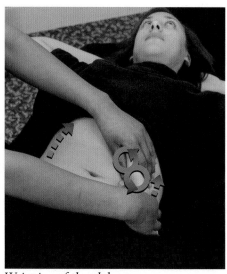

Wringing of the abdomen

One-handed muscle rolling of the quadriceps and abductors

Stance   Forward lunge stance

Hand position   Refer to table (page 119)

Technique   Using one hand, lift the muscle tissue with the fingers and roll the thumb around and down. Move the muscle away from the bone

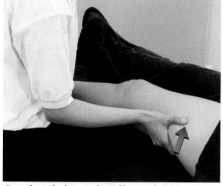

One-handed muscle rolling of the quadriceps and abductors: Step 1

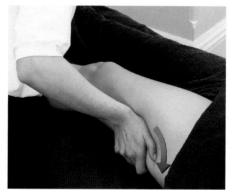

One-handed muscle rolling: Step 2

Two-handed skin rolling of the hamstrings

Stance   Stride stance

Hand position   Refer to table (page 119)

Technique   With thumbs in line, lift and grasp the muscle tissue and then push away

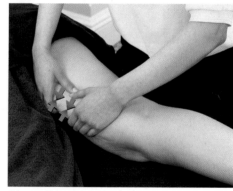

Skin rolling of the hamstrings

Alternative two-handed muscle rolling of the hamstrings

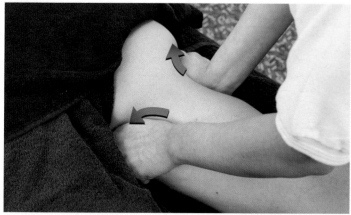

Alternative two-handed muscle rolling of the hamstrings

One-handed skin rolling of the calf

Technique	Use the same technique as in one-handed skin rolling of the quadriceps

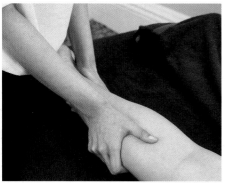

One-handed skin rolling of the calf

Skin rolling of the upper arm

Stance	Knee on the couch, supporting your client's arm on your knee
Technique	Use the same technique as in one-handed skin rolling of the quadriceps

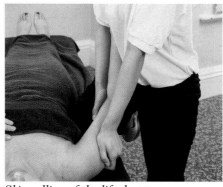

Skin rolling of the lifted upper arm

Knuckle roll of the neck

Stance	Stand behind your client's chair
Hand position	Hold the neck between the knuckles
Technique	Move the knuckles up and around the area. Apply deep pressure to the trapezius and the sternocleidomastoid muscle

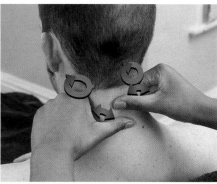

Knuckle roll of the neck

Thumb clasp of the neck

Stance	The same as in knuckle roll of the neck
Hand position	Hold the muscle tissue of the neck between the thumb and index finger
Technique	Use the thumb and index finger to apply deep upward and circular strokes

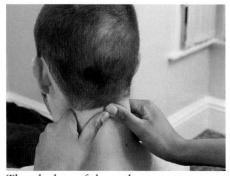

Thumb clasp of the neck

Two-handed skin rolling of the back

Technique	Use the same technique as in two-handed skin rolling of the hamstrings. With thumbs in line (parallel) to the index fingers roll, the tissue between them

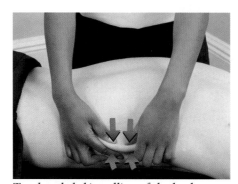

Two-handed skin rolling of the back

One-handed muscle rolling of the latissimus dorsi

Technique	Use the same technique as in one-handed muscle rolling of the quadriceps. Using four fingers to lift the tissue, roll the tissue away with the distal part of the thumb

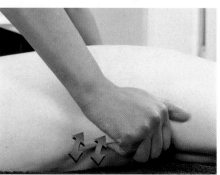

One-handed muscle rolling of the latissimus dorsi

Pummelling of the hamstrings

Stance	Forward
Hand position	Refer to table (page 119)
Technique	Using a tightly clenched fist to pummel the tissue, ensure that the hand is lifted before the next circular action takes place

Pummelling of the calf

Stance	Knee on the couch, supporting your client's leg
Technique	Use the same technique as in pummelling of the hamstrings. Support the foot with the other hand

Pummelling of the chest

Stance	Forward and then change to stride stance
Hand position	Refer to table (page 119)
Technique	Use the same technique as in pummelling the hamstring but use one hand only

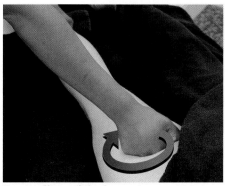
Pummelling of the hamstrings

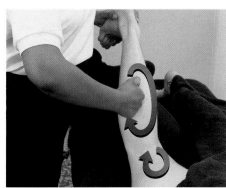
Pummelling of the calf

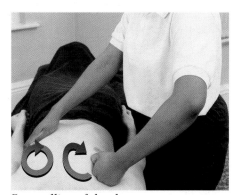
Pummelling of the chest

Pummelling of the neck

Stance	Forward, leaning over your client
Hand position	One-handed technique
Technique	Use the flat surface of the clenched fist, not the knuckles

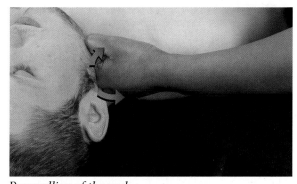
Pummelling of the neck

Pummelling of the back

Stance	Adjacent to your client
Hand position	Refer to table (page 119)
Technique	Use the same technique as in pummelling of the neck

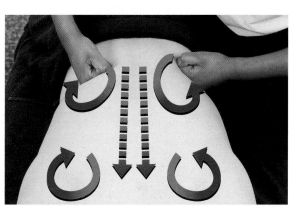
Pummelling of the back

Knuckling of the quadriceps

Stance   Forward, facing your client

Hand position Refer to table (page 119)

Technique Using the knuckles of a loosely clenched fist, work towards the heart in a circular motion. Apply moderate to deep pressure. Complete the circular motion before lifting the hand and moving on to the next part of the muscle tissue

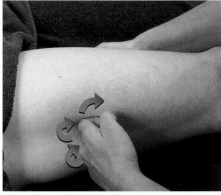

Knuckling of the quadriceps

Knuckling of the adductors

Stance   Knee supports your client's leg; client's leg is in a flexed and adducted position

Hand position Refer to table (page 119)

Technique Knuckling with the index and middle knuckles. Apply pressure in a circular motion; twisting action comes from the wrist

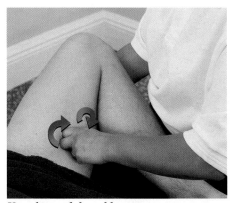

Knucking of the adductors

Knuckling of the hamstrings

Stance   Forward; client's leg is either supported by the therapist or laid flat, supported by bolsters under the foot

Hand position Refer to table (page 119)

Technique Use the same technique as in knuckling of the adductors (inner thigh)

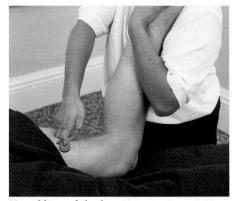

Knuckling of the hamstrings

Knuckling of the chest

Stance   Behind your client

Hand position Refer to table (page 119)

Technique 'Run' or 'walk' the knuckles across the chest. Apply moderate pressure to the chest region

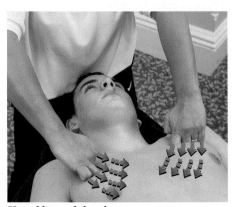

Knuckling of the chest

Knuckling of the neck

Stance	Facing your client
Hand position	Refer to table (page 119)
Technique	Use the same technique as in knuckling of the adductors (inner thigh)

Knuckling of the erector spinae (with a bent knuckle)

Stance	Adjacent to your client
Hand position	Use the index finger knuckle
Technique	Use the bent knuckle in a circular motion. The motion is a continuous circular movement up towards the head along the erector spinae. It can be used as part of a deep massage

Stroking of the quadriceps (superficial)

Stance	Forward lunge
Hand position	Use the whole palmar surface
Technique	Use the palmar surface of the hand in an upward sweeping motion. Lightly stroke the muscle tissue

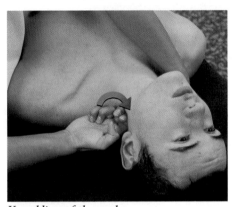

Knuckling of the neck

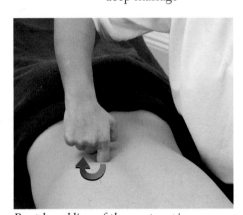

Bent knuckling of the erector spinae

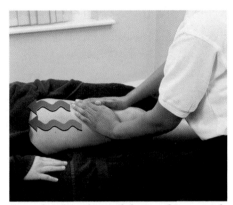

Superficial stroking of the quadriceps with the palm of the hand

Stroking of the hamstrings (deep)

Stance	Forward lunge
Hand position	Reinforced hand technique
Technique	Use the same technique as in stroking of the quadriceps (superficial). The pressure is applied through the top hand reinforcing the stroke

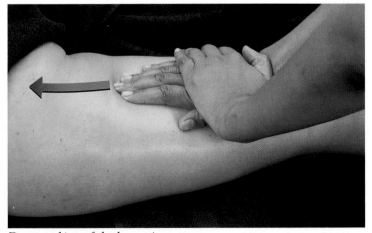

Deep stroking of the hamstrings

Stroking of the hamstrings (with the heel of the hand)

Stance   Forward lunge

Hand position   Refer to table (page 119)

Technique   Using the fingers pulled back, reinforce the hand, applying the pressure throughout the stroke

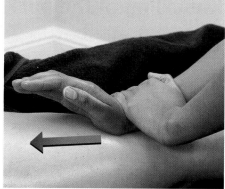

Deep stroking of the hamstrings with the heel of the hand

Forearm stroking of the calf

Stance   Forward lunge, using the body weight

Hand position   Forearm

Technique   Using the ulnar border of the forearm. Apply upward strokes to the muscle tissue

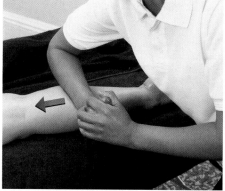

Stroking the calf with the forearm

Digital stroking of the calf

Stance   Forward lunge

Hand position   Refer to table (page 119)

Technique   Using the pads of the fingers, apply pressure in an upward motion

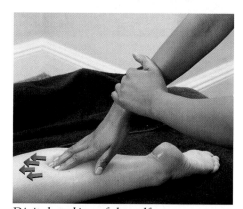

Digital stroking of the calf

Deep stroking of the trapezius

Stance   Side on to your client

Hand position   Support the wrist using the surface of the fingers

Technique   Stroke the muscle tissue with the surface of the fingers. Fingers must be spread. Complete one stroke, lift hand and return to the start for the next stroke

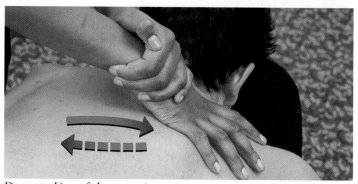

Deep stroking of the trapezius

Deep transverse stroking of the rhomboids (with the heel of the right hand)

Stance	Face your client's feet or head
Hand position	Heel of the hand (other hand supporting body)
Technique	This stroke can be applied using one or two hands. The strokes must be applied using the heel of the hand across the direction of the muscle fibres to separate the fibres

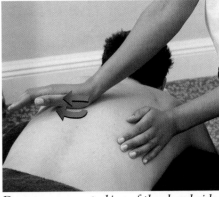

Deep transverse stroking of the rhomboids with the heel of one hand

Stroking alongside the Achilles tendon

Stance	By your client's feet
Technique	Your client's feet must slightly hang over the edge of the bed in order for the Achilles tendon to be stretched. Press against the ball of your client's feet with your thigh to maintain the stretch. Using the index and middle finger, stroke alongside the Achilles tendon in an upward motion

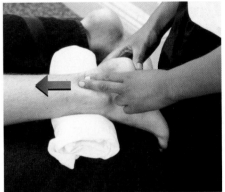

Stroking along the Achilles tendon

Stroking of the upper arm (thumbs)

Stance	Facing your client
Hand position	This will vary due to the area and size being massaged
Technique	Supporting your client's arm on your knee, use sweeping, stroking movements with the pad of the thumb

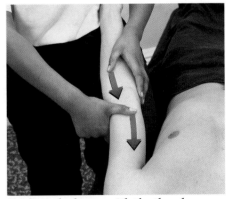

Stroking the biceps with the thumbs

Stroking the triceps (with the heel of the hand)

Stance	Adjacent to your client
Hand position	Refer to table (page 119)
Technique	Place your client's arm across his or her body; use the heel of the hand in an upward motion to apply pressure to the triceps

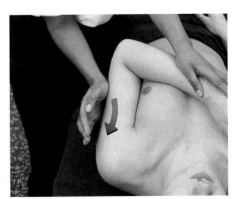

Stroking the triceps with the heel of the hand

Stroking of the chest

Stance   Head of the couch

Hand position   Refer to table (page 119)

Technique   Use the palmar surface of the hands to stroke in an upward and outward movement. Can also be performed with the digits.

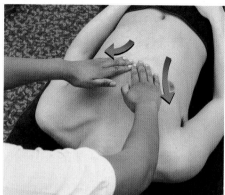

Digital stroking of the chest from sternum to shoulder

Stroking of the back (with the elbow)

Stance   Side on to your client

Hand position   Elbow flexed and supported by the other hand

Technique   Use slow upward stroking movements. At the end of each stroke, lift the elbow from the area and return to the first phase of the technique and repeat

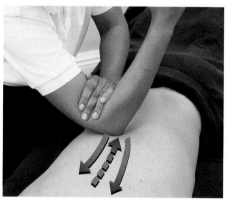

Deep stroking of the erector spinae with the elbow

Digital stroking of the neck

Stance   Behind your client

Hand position   Support your client's neck using the thumbs

Technique   Sweep the hands up towards the head. This technique can be used with either superficial or deep pressure

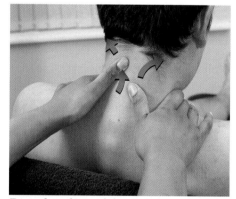

Digital stroking of the neck

Hacking of the gluteals (two-handed)

Stance   Stride

Hand position   Refer to table (page 119)

Technique   Using both hands together, strike the muscle tissue. Use this technique in areas of large muscle tissue

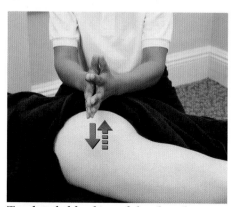

Two-handed hacking of the gluteals

Single hacking of the gluteals

Stance	Stride
Hand position	Palms parallel, facing each other
Technique	Make contact with the muscle tissue with the little and ring fingers. Strike the area being treated with both hands alternately

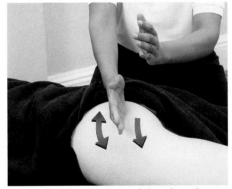

Single-handed hacking of the gluteals

Cupping of the hamstrings

Stance	Stride
Hand position	Refer to table (page 119)
Technique	With both hands strike the area alternately. Contact of the hands on the treated area should produce a hollow sound

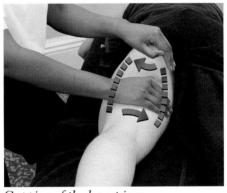

Cupping of the hamstrings

Pounding of the gluteals

Stance	Stride
Hand position	Refer to table (page 119)
Technique	While rolling the hands over each other, strike the muscle tissue using the ulnar borders of the hands

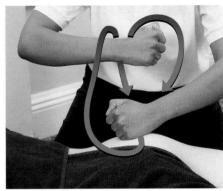

Pounding the gluteals

Slapping of the hamstrings

Stance	Stride
Hand position	Refer to table (page 119)
Technique	Hold hands flat and strike the area with both hands alternately

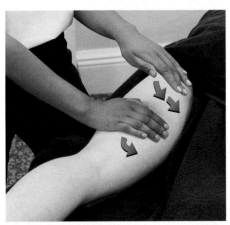

Slapping the hamstrings

Beating of the gluteals

Stance	Stride
Hand position	Refer to table (page 119)
Technique	Use the knuckles in a horizontal position

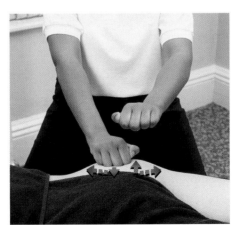

Beating the gluteals with the knuckles

Beating of the hamstrings

Stance	Stride
Hand position	Refer to table (page 119)
Technique	Use the ulnar borders of the fists in a vertical position

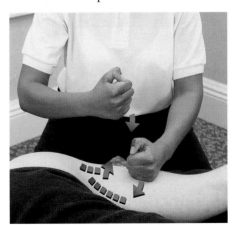

Beating the hamstrings with the fists

Effleurage of the abdominals

Stance Forward

Hand position Palmar stroking

Technique Start this technique from the bikini line, performing an upward stroke over the rectus abdominus and then move outwards towards the obliques. Use the same line on the return phase but release the pressure

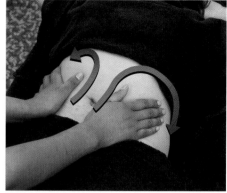

Effleurage of the abdominals

Kneading the gluteals

Stance Side on to your client

Hand position Refer to table (page 119)

Technique Compress the tissue between two hands alternately

Finger circle of the neck

Stance Behind client

Hand position One-handed technique

Technique Use the pads of the fingers of one hand and apply pressure in a circular motion

Thumb frictions of the Achilles tendon

Stance Adjacent to foot

Hand position Clasp the Achilles tendon between the thumb and index finger

Technique Exert deep pressure between the thumb and index finger while moving the Achilles tendon

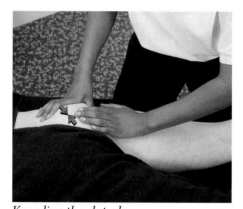

Kneading the gluteals

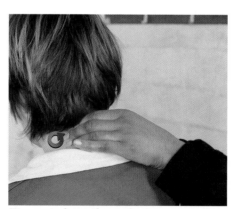

Finger circle on the neck

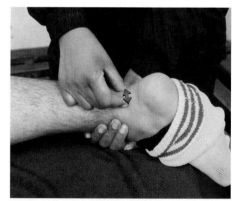

Thumb frictions of the Achilles tendon

Digital friction of the calf

Stance At foot of bed

Hand position Refer to table (page 119)

Technique Using a reinforced finger, apply friction to the area where the trauma has been located. The movement is small, deep and precise. Move the fingers back and forth over this area

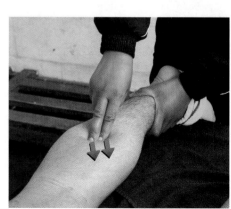

Digital frictions of the calf

Transverse frictions on erector spinae

Technique Locate the trauma. Place the index and middle fingers either side of the trauma. Use the reinforced friction technique transversely across the muscle tissue in order to separate the muscle fibres and loosen any adhesions

Stretching the hamstrings on the couch

Technique Client with bent leg resting on couch. Support opposite leg and move it towards client's chest. Hold at point of resistance

Stretching the quadriceps on the couch

Technique Push the hips into the couch. Move the heel of the foot towards the gluteals, flexing at the knee

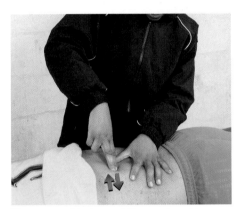

Transverse frictions of the erector spinae

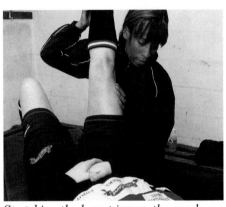

Stretching the hamstring on the couch

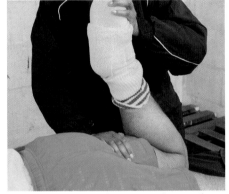

Stretching the quadriceps on the couch

Heel (of the hand) squeeze

Technique Clasp hands together and compress belly of the muscle together

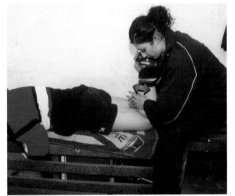

Heel squeeze on the calf in the changing room

Palmar kneading of the quadriceps in a changing room environment

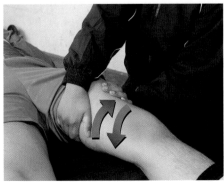

Transverse palmar kneading of the quadriceps

▶ **KNOWLEDGE CHECK**

1 Which muscles are involved in effluraging the front and back of the leg?

2 Which muscles are involved in effluraging the arm?

3 Which muscles are involved in effluraging the back?

4 What are the benefits of wringing?

5 Which muscles are involved in wringing the hamstrings?

6 When might you use knuckling in sports massage?

7 Name the muscles of the neck.

8 How would you perform deep stroking of the trapezius?

9 What effect will tapotement have on the body?

10 What are the benefits of using frictions in sports massage?

Event
massage

Sports massage is used by many people who frequently participate in sport; it can be effective before, during and after a training session, competition or sporting activity. In these instances it is known as pre-event massage, inter-event massage, and post-event massage.

Pre-event massage

Before an event or activity massaging the major muscles which are to be used will help an athlete to prepare for the challenge ahead both physically and psychologically. A pre-event massage can be performed a few minutes or hours before the athlete is due to compete or it can be performed in the days leading up to the event as part of the athlete's training programme. The aims of the massage and the techniques, depth and pressure used will vary depending on when the pre-event massage is performed.

General aims of pre-event massage

The general aims of pre-event massage are to:

- raise the core temperature of the muscles, thus helping the athlete to warm up
- stretch the tissues – mainly to minimize injury and maximize performance
- increase range of movement, improve joint mobility and blood circulation
- prepare the athlete both physically and psychologically before a sporting event.

Raising the core temperature of the muscles

Muscles that are warm tend to 'work' better and allow the athlete to perform better, so a massage usually begins with an effleurage; this involves stroking the muscle tissue in a specific way, to increase the blood flow to the area, thereby producing heat and raising the core temperature of the muscles. The increased flow of oxygenated blood to the area will bring with it nutrients which feed the muscle tissue, and also any waste products present will be taken away.

A pre-event massage should target the main muscle groups that are to be used. However, the techniques used, depth and pressure will vary according to:

- the needs of your client
- the competition/activity
- muscle size
- time available.

Stretching of the muscle tissue

Massage can help to stretch muscle fibres and minimize the risk of injury. Thumb sliding and muscle rolling, kneading and wringing are some of the techniques that can increase the flexibility of the tissues, which will allow the muscles to work efficiently. These techniques can be used in both pre-event and post-event massage.

> **! MASSAGE FACT**
>
> Never perform a deep massage in the minutes or hours leading up to an event or activity. The massage must be performed with a moderate pressure, so as not to relax the muscles totally.

Increasing the range of movement and improve mobility and flexibility

Each joint in the body has its own natural range of movement. Flexibility training can help to increase the mobility of a joint, thus increasing the range of movement. If, for some reason, mobility is inhibited, then the functioning of the muscles will be affected, which will result in a loss of range of movement. Friction massage around joints, performed using the thumb or fingers, can help to break down or loosen adhesions, which may inhibit mobility.

Muscle tension will affect the flexibility of the muscles. The tenser the muscle is, the harder it will be to stretch it. Massage can help to reduce muscle tension and encourage 'muscle relaxation', thus enabling the athlete to incorporate effective flexibility stretching into their regime.

> **! PRE-EVENT FACT**
>
> A pre-event massage should never induce total relaxation, which may result in sleep. An athlete needs to be prepared to compete and should remain focused throughout the treatment. Massage can help an athlete to remain calm but focused and able to concentrate on the event ahead.

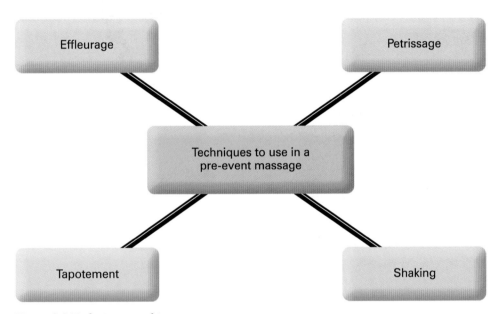

Figure 8.1 *Techniques used in a pre-event massage*

Preparing the athlete before a sporting event

As well as physically preparing the muscles before an event, massage can also help the athlete to mentally relax and focus on the event in hand.

The following examples demonstrate techniques that could be used in a pre-event massage. The techniques that you choose will depend upon your client's needs, the major muscles being used, the needs of the sport, and the position in which he or she plays.

Note: some techniques listed in the examples below are descibed in the chapter 'Advanced techniques in sports massage'.

> **! MASSAGE FACT**
>
> A massage should never be used in place of a physical warm-up; an athlete, sports person or competitor should ensure that they undertake a full thorough warm-up and effective and sufficient stretching.

An example of a ten-minute pre-event massage

Client: Rugby player, full back

Treatment: Pre-event massage

Key areas: Legs

Notes:

- ☐ Client lying in supine position.
- ☐ Place bolsters under the knee and ankle joint.

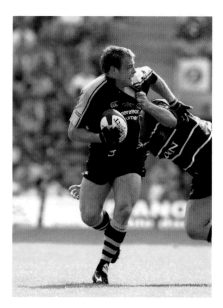

Front of legs

1 Effleurage of whole leg
2 Effleurage of thigh
3 Wringing of inner thigh
4 Palmar kneading of thigh
5 Hacking of thigh
6 Effleurage of whole leg to knee
7 Thumb circles around knee joint
8 Effleurage of lower leg
9 Effleurage of whole leg to finish.

Back of legs

Notes:

- ☐ Client lying in prone position.
- ☐ Place bolsters under the foot/ankle.

1 Effleurage of whole leg
2 Effleurage of hamstrings
3 Palmar kneading of hamstrings
4 Knuckle twist of hamstrings
5 Wringing of hamstrings
6 Hacking of hamstrings
7 Effleurage of hamstrings
8 Pounding of top and side of hamstrings
9 Effleurage of hamstrings
10 Large thumb circles over hamstrings
11 Muscle rolling of hamstrings
12 Wringing of calf
13 Kneading of calf
14 Hacking of calf
15 Effleurage of whole leg.

Example of a ten- to fifteen-minute pre-event massage

Client: Javelin thrower

Treatment: Pre-event massage

Key areas: Arms, back

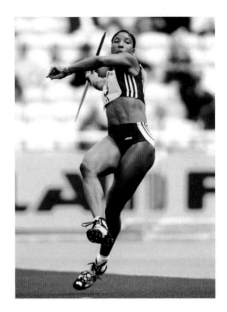

Arms

Notes:

☐ Effleurage of the arm can be performed when your client is in an upright or supine position.

☐ Support the arm with your other hand or rest it on your thigh/knee for stability.

1 Effleurage of arm from palm to shoulder
2 Effleurage of upper arm
3 Finger circles around the shoulder joint
4 One-handed kneading of upper arm
5 One-handed knuckling of triceps and biceps
6 Effleurage of upper arm
7 Circumduction of shoulder (forward and backward)
8 Shaking of biceps and triceps
9 Thumb circles over forearm
10 Thumb circles around wrist
11 Mobilization of the wrist (flexion and extension)
12 Effleurage of whole arm.

Back

Notes:

☐ Client in the prone position.

☐ Client may need support or may feel comfortable with a towel placed under the abdomen.

☐ Be selective with the strokes you choose to use as your client may be feeling pain or may have areas of tenderness.

1 Effleurage of the back from the sacrum to the deltoids
2 Kneading of the back
3 Wringing of the latissimus dorsi
4 Kneading around the scapula
5 Thumb circles along the erector spinae
6 Knuckling along the erector spinae
7 Effleurage of the trapezius
8 Kneading of the trapezius
9 Effleurage of whole back.

Post-event massage

After an event, competition or physical activity, it is important that the athlete allows the body to recover from the stress that has been placed upon it. The recovery process of an athlete after an event or training will usually start with a physical cool-down, performing a series of exercises, which will gradually reduce the heart rate, and effective stretching to reduce the risk of muscle soreness.

A post-event massage can be performed instead of or after a physical cool-down and can last from anything between ten and 60 minutes. The therapist, using effleurage, stroking and petrissage techniques, can help the muscles recover after strenuous activity. It is, however, recommended that athletes try and incorporate cool-down activities into their training programme and use massage afterwards. A lot of athletes who work hard during training or competitions do not manage to perform a physical cool-down, so massage can be beneficial and effective in the removal of waste products.

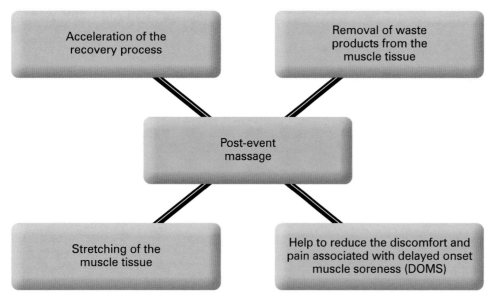

Figure 8.2 Benefits of post-event massage

Removal of waste products from the muscle tissue

When muscles have had a lot of stress placed upon them through exercise, an event or competition, there will be an increase in waste products in the muscle tissue, which may cause soreness and stiffness. Techniques such as effleurage, stroking and petrissage will help to increase the flow of oxygen-rich blood to the muscle, which in turn will transport the waste products away. They will also relax the muscle tissue.

Acceleration of the recovery process

Massage helps to speed up the recovery process of an athlete after exercise, an event or competition by helping to rid the muscles of the accumulation of waste products, thus helping him or her to recover from muscle fatigue. If an athlete does not have sufficient time to recover from an event or prolonged intense training, then a noticeable difference may be evident in his or her next performance. Massage will help to reduce muscle soreness, muscle fatigue and reduce the likelihood of injuries occurring or reoccurring.

Massage can also help to speed up the recovery process of an athlete after the acute phase of an injury. Soft tissue injuries (tendons, ligaments, muscle, skin) usually occur as a result of over-training without adequate rest periods, poor technique, or as a result of excessive stresses being placed upon the specific parts.

The aim of massage after injury is to help restore full function to muscles, ligaments and tendons. At this stage, light massage techniques, such as effleurage, stroking and petrissage, can also help to reduce pain.

Stretching of the muscle tissue

During a post-event massage and pre-event massage, the main muscles used by the athlete can be stretched in a number of ways:

- static stretching
- dynamic or ballistic stretching (not recommended but still used in sports such as karate, ballet and gymnastics)
- PNF (proprioceptive neuromuscular facilitation)

Detailed descriptions of these stretching methods are given on pages 146–8.

Reduction of the discomfort and pain associated with DOMS

Delayed-onset muscle soreness, or DOMS, is a soreness that occurs in the exercised muscles or joints for up to two days after excessive training, competition or activity. It is not known exactly how DOMS occurs. It is *not* thought to be caused by a build-up of lactic acid, but by a number of factors which include muscle spasm, minute tearing within the muscle tissue, inflammation or overstretching. Massage after activity, however, will help to reduce pain, stiffness and discomfort.

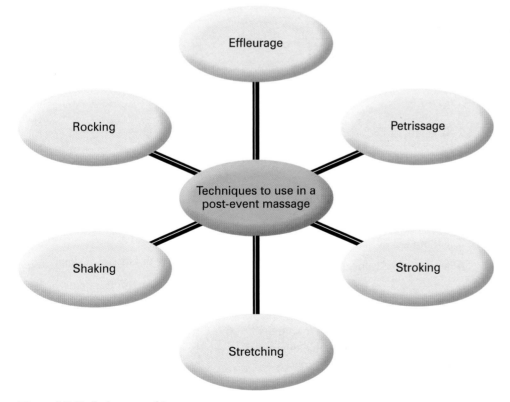

Figure 8.3 Techniques used in a post-event massage

Example of a 45-minute post-event massage

Client: Basketball player

Treatment: Post-event massage   **Key areas:** Legs, arms, back

Notes:

☐ Slow, rhythmical strokes.

☐ Ask your client if the pressure is suitable or painful while you are treating him or her.

Front of legs

1 Effleurage of whole leg (feet to hip)
2 Effleurage of thigh
3 Transverse palmar kneading of thigh
4 Wringing of adductor muscles
5 Wringing of quadriceps
6 Muscle rolling of upper thigh
7 Effleurage of upper thigh
8 Slow stroking of upper thigh – palm
9 Slow stroking of upper thigh – forearm
10 Effleurage of upper thigh
11 Thumb sliding around the knee
12 Effleurage of lower leg
13 Passive stretching of hamstrings.

Back of legs

1 Effleurage of ankle to hip
2 Effleurage of hamstrings
3 Kneading of hamstrings
4 Stroking of hamstrings – palm
5 Circular stroking of hamstrings – heel of the hand
6 Stroking of hamstrings – digits
7 Effleurage from hamstrings to calf
8 Stroking from ankles to top calf – palm
9 Thumb circles
10 Stroking of calf – heel of hand
11 Thumb sliding of calf
12 Effleurage of calf
13 Kneading of calf

14 Wringing of calf
15 Effleurage of calf
16 Finger kneading of Achilles tendon
17 Effleurage of whole leg
18 Passive stretch of quadriceps.

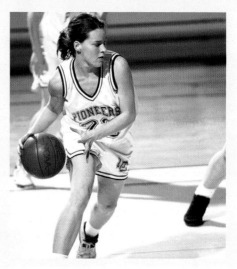

Arms

1 Effleurage of arms
2 Effleurage of biceps and triceps
3 Stroking of triceps – heel of hand
4 Stroking of biceps – digits
5 Effleurage of triceps and biceps
6 Kneading of biceps and triceps – heel of hand
7 Effleurage of whole arm
8 Stroking of forearm – palm
9 Finger circles over forearm.

Back

1 Rocking of back
2 Effleurage of back
3 Stroking of back – digits
4 Reinforced circular stroking around scapula
5 Effleurage of back
6 Kneading of trapezius
7 Effleurage of back
8 Kneading of trapezius
9 Effleurage of back

10 Bent knuckling along the erector spinae
11 Effleurage of back
12 Large thumb circles along the erector spinae
13 Effleurage of back
14 Wringing of latissimus dorsi
15 Deep stroking of trapezius
16 Effleurage of back
17 Cross-fibre stretch
18 Effleurage.

Note that the amount of time spent on each technique will vary with the needs of your client, the aims of the massage, and the time available.

Inter-event massage

Inter-event massage is performed during a series of activities; for example, an athlete performing in the heptathlon may have a massage in between the different events to isolate and prepare individual muscles for the different activities. An inter-event massage can also be performed at half-time during football or other sports matches. This will:

☐ maintain body temperature
☐ relieve muscle tension
☐ prepare the major muscles to be used in the second half.

In these instances, the massage might last from anything between three and ten minutes, or up to 25 minutes, depending on each individual situation. Effleurage, petrissage and some tapotement can be used during an inter-event massage. However, if muscle soreness is present, then avoid using techniques such as tapotement on sensitive areas, as these may cause further pain or discomfort to the athlete.

Example of a three- to five-minute stimulating inter-event massage

Client: Gymnast between apparatus

Treatment: Inter-event massage

Notes:

☐ Massage the main muscles which are going to be used and those used in the previous event.
☐ Perform the massage at moderate speed and moderate pressure.
☐ Stimulating techniques such as tapotement may be required; however, the techniques of a post-event massage may be required instead to aid the recovery process.

Front of legs	Back of legs
1 Effleurage of whole leg	**1** Effleurage of whole leg
2 Effleurage of quadriceps	**2** Effleurage of hamstrings
3 Wringing of quadriceps	**3** Wringing of hamstrings
4 Hacking	**4** Hacking
5 Cupping	**5** Cupping
6 Effleurage	**6** Effleurage
7 Passive stretching.	**7** Passive stretching.

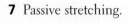

► KNOWLEDGE CHECK

1 Explain the effects that a pre-event massage would have on an athlete preparing for a competition.

2 What is post-event massage?

3 How is post-event massage of value to a sports person?

4 Which type of massage movements do you think should be used in a post-event massage and why?

5 In general terms, how would an athlete benefit from incorporating sports massage into their training schedule?

6 Which techniques would you not use in a post-event massage and why?

7 What causes muscle fatigue?

8 How does massage assist in treating muscle fatigue?

9 Which four factors govern the type of pressure used in massage.

Appendix: Stretching

Muscle tissue is joined to bone by connective tissue called tendons, and bones are connected to other bones by ligaments. Because of this, it is important to understand the property of connective tissue when discussing flexibility. Connective tissue is composed of a matrix of non-living cells that give it the ability to withstand great tension, weight and trauma.

Flexibility is often a neglected component of fitness. It can be described as a range of movements around a joint or series of joints. By contrast, stretches are the individual exercises that help to improve flexibility.

Before carrying out stretching techniques on a client, it is essential for the therapist to be fully aware of the correct procedures, to avoid damage to muscles, their connective tissue and attachments.

There are various reasons for performing flexibility exercises during a therapy session: to test the range of movement, for instance, and to help to design a flexibility programme. There is a difference between stretches testing for flexibility in a therapy session and those used when as part of the warm-up and cool-down of a training session.

The stretches used in a warm-up are to prepare the muscle groups that will be used in performance. The stretches used in a cool-down are primarily for relaxation and the reduction of muscle soreness after performance. When used as part of a flexibility training session, flexibility exercises aim to increase the range of movement around a joint or series of joints.

It is vitally important to have a balance of flexibility over the whole body to help reduce the risk of injury. Lack of flexibility during movement of one area may lead to increased flexibility of other areas or compensation for the lack of flexibility, causing long-term damage.

There are various factors that can affect the range of motion around a joint. These include the following.

- The type of joint determines the type of movement. For example, the hinge joint found in the knee can only perform movements of flexion and extension. If an attempt is made to make the joint perform a rotating movement, then the knee joint is at risk of damage.
- The condition of the muscles and other soft tissues can help or hinder the range of movement of a joint. If stretching takes place, the elasticity of the muscle tissue is increased before contraction is performed. This increased elasticity reduces the amount of resistance that the muscle has to the movement and will reduce the risk of damage to the joint structure.
- The local temperature of the body's tissues can help or hinder the range of movement of a joint. For example, an increase in local temperature increases mobility by decreasing the density of synovial fluid around the joint and increasing the flexibilty of the connective tissue of the muscle, making the ligaments and tendons more workable.
- The age and gender of an individual affects his or her mobility and the flexibility of his or her muscles. As age increases, mobility and flexibility decrease. This process can be delayed if regular flexibility exercises are carried out. The optimum time to develop flexibility is during the early developmental years, as the calcification of the bones is not fully completed. Therefore, flexibility exercises during these years helps to increase elastic properties around the joints. Females are more flexible than males after the pubescent years.

! STRETCH FACT

Stretching of the muscle fascia, muscles and tendons can be achieved through massage. Ligaments cannot be stretched because they are non-elastic.

! STRETCH FACT

Stretching can help to reduce muscle tension.

There are different methods of stretching for flexibility:

- static
- dynamic
- proprioceptive neuromuscular facilitation (PNF).

Maintenance stretches are held for 6 to 20 seconds, usually during a warm-up, as part of a training or competitive session. Developmental stretches are usually held for 15 to 30 seconds during the cool-down section of performance.

Static flexibility stretching

Static flexibility stretching is the slow, sustained stretch of a joint. It lengthens the muscle tissue and is held in position for a few moments. The slow movements during this method of stretching allow information to be passed to the brain, which then triggers a stretch reflex to resist the stretch. Holding the stretch for approximately ten seconds allows the area to become less sensitive to the stretch, resulting in the muscle tissues being stretched without damage.

Static flexibility stretching is divided into two categories: active or passive stretches.

- Active stretching is where a muscle is lengthened in a position without assistance but requires the strength of other muscles to hold the position.
- Passive stretching is where a muscle group is assisted throughout the stretch by an external force such as a partner, physical object or gravity.

The static method of stretching requires a muscle to be thoroughly warm and relaxed. The antagonistic muscle needs to be pulled towards its target very slowly and to its limit. Holding the stretch is essential before increasing the stretch beyond this point for the full benefits to be experienced. The stretch must be held for at least six seconds for the golgi tendons to respond. The golgi tendons override the original stretch receptor response to allow a greater stretch of the muscle. This helps the contracted muscle to relax and reduces the tension during the stretch.

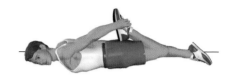
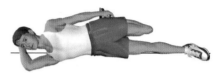

Figure 8.4 Front of thigh stretch (lying)

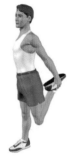

Figure 8.5 Front of thigh stretch

Figure 8.6 Back of thigh stretch

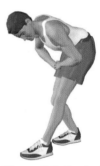
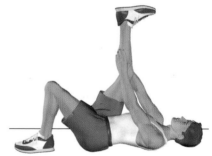

Figure 8.7 Back of thigh stretch (lying)

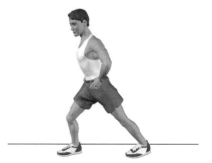

Figure 8.8 Calf stretch

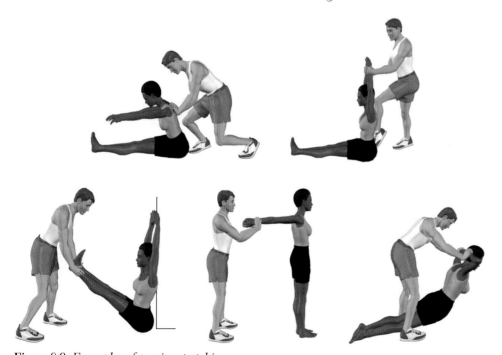

Figure 8.9 Examples of passive stretching

Dynamic flexibility stretching

Dynamic flexibility stretching includes stretches that are commonly known as ballistic stretches. These are performed during a fast, bouncing action where the momentum of body weight assists in taking the joint beyond its range of movement. Ballistic stretching has caused concern due to the high risk of injury to the muscle group being stretched. It is not generally recommended but is still used in specific sports, such as dance and karate, to obtain a greater range of motion around a joint area during movement.

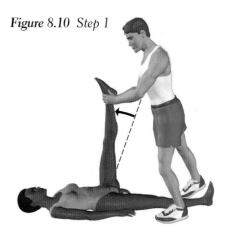

Figure 8.10 Step 1

Proprioceptive neuromuscular facilitation (PNF)

This method of stretching is classed as an advanced form of stretching and can be dangerous if not performed using the correct technique. It is during these types of stretches that the therapist must fully understand the procedure to assist in the movements with the client. If pain and burning sensations are experienced, signals are being sent that damage has occurred or is about to occur.

As with many types of flexibility stretching methods, PNF can be categorized as active or passive.

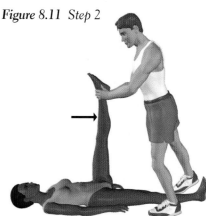

Figure 8.11 Step 2

Passive PNF

1 The therapist flexes the client's leg at the hip joint until slight discomfort is felt.

2 The client pushes against the therapist's resistance by contracting the position. This position is held for approximately ten seconds.

3 The client relaxes the leg for ten seconds but holds the position of the leg being stretched.

4 The client attempts a comncentric contraction (contraction through the shortening of the muscle) of the hip flexors.

Active PNF

1 The therapist flexes the client's leg at the hip joint until slight discomfort is felt.

2 The client pushes against the therapist's resistance by contracting the hip flexors. This position is held for approximately ten seconds.

3 The client relaxes the leg for ten seconds.

4 The client attempts a concentric contraction (contraction through the shortening of the muscle) of the hip flexors.

5 The client then relaxes.

6 The therapist applies further passive pressure, where the client's leg would have moved to a position of increased angle at the hip joint.

7 Repeat step 2 of the procedure.

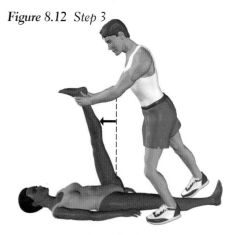

Figure 8.12 Step 3

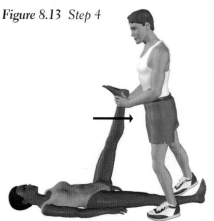

Figure 8.13 Step 4

- Palpation
- Vibrations
- Frictions
- Strain counter strain
- Neuromuscular technique
- Muscle energy technique

Advanced techniques used in

sports massage

Palpation

Palpation is an exploratory technique whereby the therapist slowly glides his or her hands over structures in order to examine them. The pads of the fingers or thumbs are used to feel individual muscles, or groups of muscles, to assess the condition of the tissue in order to identify any irregularities.

Palpation is a skill that requires continuous practice and you must have a good knowledge of anatomy and physiology in order to identify what is being felt. As soon as you place your fingers or thumb on your client, you should note the temperature of his or her skin. Whilst palpating, it is important to observe your client's reaction to your touch. Watch his or her facial expression – does your client move or twitch when you touch a specific area? Does he or she gasp when pain is felt? Do not be afraid to talk to your client as you are palpating; this will allow you to gather further information.

It is important to note that there are areas in the body where **trigger points** are found; these are painful areas within the muscle tissue that feel tender, and can sometimes feel very painful, when touched. When trigger points are touched during massage or palpation, pain is usually felt somewhere else in the body. This is known as referred pain. The aim of performing massage where trigger points are found is to reduce the effect of the referred pain and to restore the full function of the muscle tissue. Direct pressure or frictions are effective in helping to reduce the pain, direct pressure being applied by means of the pads of the fingers or thumb or by means of the elbow. An even pressure should be applied and held for ten to twenty seconds. At the end of the treatment, take your client through a range of stretches for each muscle being treated; use passive stretching and ensure that full-range movements are used.

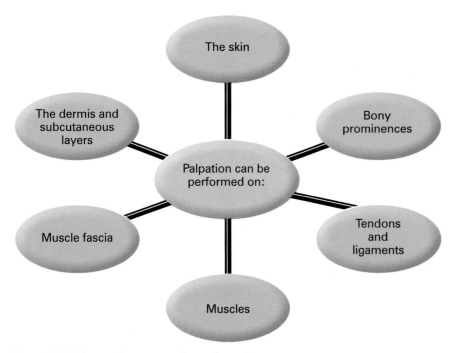

Figure 9.2 Where palpation can be performed

NB Palpation should not be performed without adequate training and a thorough understanding of anatomy and physiology.

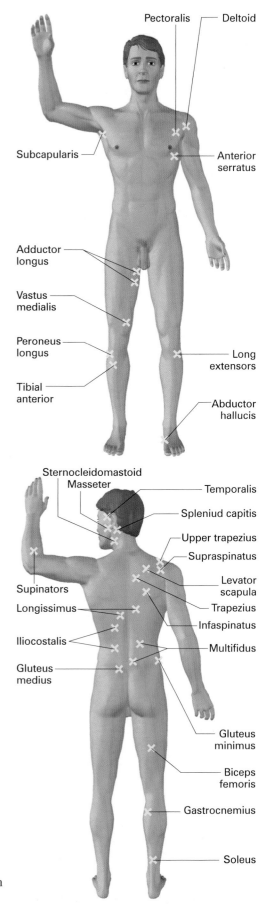

Figure 9.1 The body's common trigger poin

Vibrations

Vibrations can be performed using one or both hands and using one, two or all of the fingers. The fingers are shaken in a fast trembling action, which is transferred to the body part being worked on with a moderate degree of pressure. There are two types of vibrations: static and running.

Static vibrations

These are applied using the pads of the fingers and thumbs and also the balls of the fingertips, which are placed on a nerve centre. The rapid trembling action, as described above, should be applied with the movement coming from your forearm.

Both static and running vibrations can be performed using the fingers, the thumb or the palmar surface of the hands.

Running vibrations

These are applied using the whole hand, which travels along a nerve path. The movement comes from your forearm, which contracts and relaxes while producing the trembling movement.

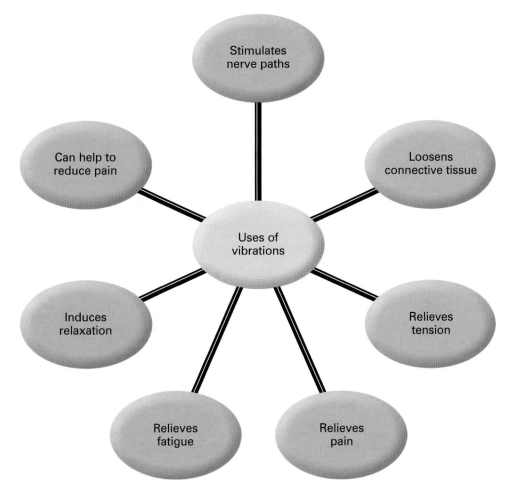

Figure 9.3   Uses of vibrations in sports massage

Frictions

Frictions are a very deep penetrative and specialized technique, which can be performed using the pads of the fingers or thumbs. This technique is frequently used in sports massage when trauma has been located in muscles, tendons or ligaments. Frictions are either performed using a small circular motion (circular frictions), or can be applied transversally across the muscle fibres (transverse frictions or cross-fibre frictions).

Frictions may be painful to your client at first, so it is always advisable to state this and suggests deep breathing through the discomfort. This assists in relieving tension.

Circular frictions

Circular frictions, as well as being applied using the pads of the fingers or thumb, can also be performed using the elbow, which can allow deep penetration of the area being worked on. Circular frictions produce a stretch-release effect on the tissues.

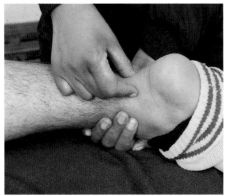

Thumb frictions of the Achilles tendon

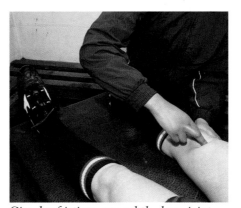

Circular frictions around the knee joint

The problem area should be isolated and circular frictions applied; these should gradually increase in depth, and focus wholly on the trauma.

Transverse frictions

1   Accurately locate the trauma using palpation.

2   Place the area to be worked on in full stretch.

3   Spread the fingers of the hand not applying the frictions around the area of trauma.

4   Locate the trauma between the index and middle fingers or the thumb and index finger and use them as a guide.

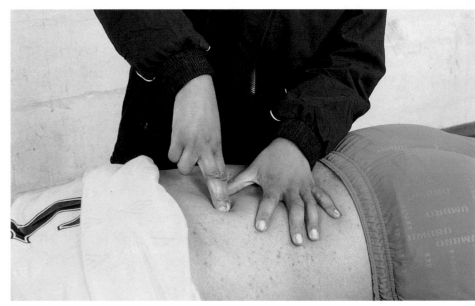

Transverse frictions of the erector spinae

5 Slowly apply the frictions transversally, at a right angle to the muscle fibres being worked on. Use the pad of the thumb or finger, or the pad of the index finger with the middle finger on top for reinforcement. The latter allows a deeper pressure to be applied.

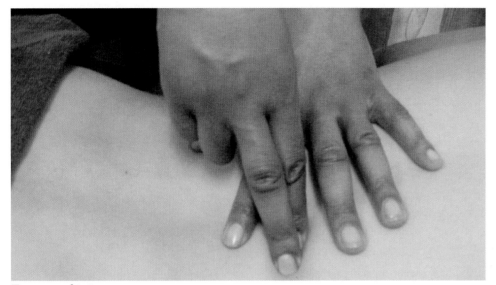

Transverse frictions

6 Apply the frictions using a back-and-forth movement. Because of the deep pressure being applied, contact with the trauma should be in spurts of one to three minutes, with a total of ten to twenty minutes per session.

7 Always massage and passively stretch the area after treatment.

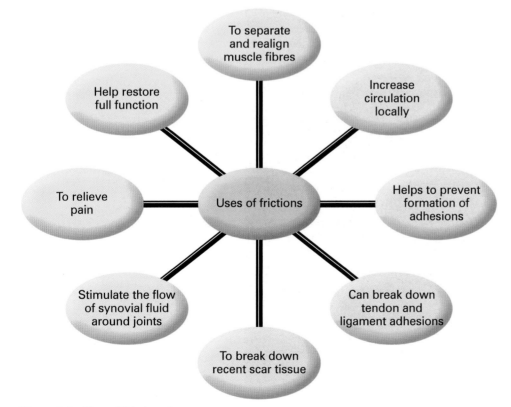

Figure 9.4   Uses of frictions in sports massage

Strain counter strain

The aim of this technique is to reduce tension or discomfort within the muscle tissue. It works by re-educating the muscle fibres so that the muscle is able to function as effectively as before the onset of the tension or discomfort.

How to perform strain counter strain

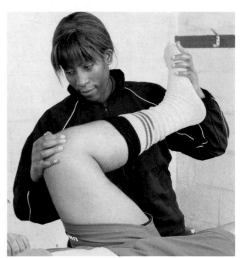

1 The area to be worked on needs to be warmed using effleurage and petrissage.

2 The length of the muscle must be shortened by passively flexing the joint. If the muscle is placed in full stretch, then your client will undoubtedly experience pain. The flexed position should be held for 90 seconds. Holding this flexed position will help to reduce any muscle spasm.

3 Slowly stretch the injured muscle passively, ensuring that your client does not initiate an isometric contraction, which would in turn become an active stretch, which could make the condition worse.

4 An improvement should be seen in the muscle length and once it has been fully restored, the position should be held for up to 60 seconds, which allows the muscles, soft tissue and nervous system to adapt.

Strain counter strain performed on the leg

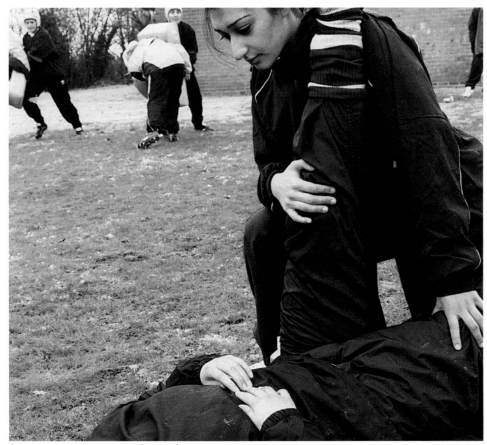

Strain counter strain on the pitch

Neuromuscular technique

The aim of this technique is to reduce tension and relieve pain. It works by inhibiting the neural message from the muscle to the central nervous system, which in turn will relieve pain, reduce tension, and relax the muscle. This technique can be applied with the pads of the fingers, thumbs, or with the elbow, and is performed during a massage session after the area has been warmed with effleurage and petrissage.

How to perform neuromuscular technique

Once the area is warm:

1 Slowly palpate and explore the area to locate the trauma or tender spot within the muscle.

2 Apply gradual pressure using the pads of the fingers or thumbs, or the elbow, for 60–90 seconds. Deep, but tolerable, pressure should be applied.

3 Inform your client that the pressure may be painful at first but that the pain should gradually fade. If the pain does not fade, then palpate and revisit the site up to three times, applying pressure for no more than 90 seconds. During this time, keep talking to your client and asking if the pain is fading.

If the pain does not fade, cross-fibre frictions may be applied to the area to try and loosen or free any adhesions that may be present within the tissue.

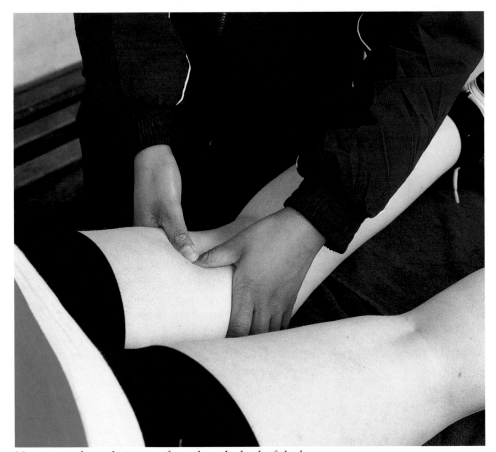

Neuromuscular technique performed on the back of the leg

Muscle energy technique (MET)

MET is a technique that uses your client's own exertion and movement as a primary force when treating a soft tissue problem. However, you must assist in the safe and correct application of the technique. MET comprises a variety of techniques. These include:

☐ stretch techniques

☐ strength techniques

☐ techniques that break down tough or fibrous adhesions.

Initially, it is important to identify weaknesses or problematic areas of the body. Your role as therapist must include developing your knowledge of the muscle groups that work together to create or maintain movement. As stated in the anatomy and physiology section, muscles work in groups; this is essential for the body to be able to move in a smooth and efficient fashion. As the agonist muscle contracts, the antagonistic muscle needs to relax. This partnership is known as reciprocal inhibition. Nerves are also involved in this process, sending impulses to the central nervous system which then relays information to reflex centres, these centres then send impulses to the antagonistic muscle group that cause them to relax. If a muscle remains tense after an activity, this sends messages to the relevant centre that the muscle is contracting. When the muscle contracts, the antagonistic muscle group needs to be in a state of relaxation. However, if a muscle has become weak through injury, then the tension or the strength of the muscle group will need to be increased by the opposing muscle. Maintaining a balance between the muscle groups is essential; therefore, if a muscle has become tense, it will need to be stretched first to allow the strength levels of the weaker opposing muscle to increase.

> **! MET FACT**
>
> You the therapist must work with your client by relaxing throughout the delivery of the technique.

Stretch techniques

MET uses two different types of stretch techniques that aim to stretch the muscle group beyond its usual capability. These techniques work on the muscle's state of relaxation.

Post-isometric relaxation (PIR)

The muscle performs an isometric contraction and is then allowed to relax for a short period of time. The muscle should become inhibited during this phase for approximately five to ten seconds; this can be classed as a deep relaxation state of the tissues where the muscle can be passively stretched further for approximately ten to fifteen seconds. Holding the muscle in these positions gives the nervous system time to transmit information to the reflex arcs so as to habituate the tissues to the new position. Moving the muscle beyond its original state can be maintained as long as stretching exercises are carried out on a regular basis and the original muscular problem has been sorted out.

Reciprocal inhibition (RI)

This technique requires your client to be well timed through the contraction, relaxation and contraction phases. The muscle performs an isometric contraction to make the antagonistic muscle group relax. Once the contraction has been completed, a further contraction takes place immediately to prevent the opposing muscle reverting back to its 'normal' muscle tone.

The benefits of MET stretch techniques are that they can help reduce tension in a muscle group and allow efficient massage to take place. The focus of these techniques is on the duration of the stretch rather than the force being applied to the area.

As therapist you put the appropriate part of your client's body in a position that will allow the muscle group being treated to be moved to a point of mild stretch (this position needs to be fixed to prevent unwanted movement during treatment). The stretch should not cause any pain to your client. The first sign of tension as the stretch is carried out is known as the barrier. You need to position your body to ensure that the muscle group remains in a state of mild stretch or tension.

MET focuses on the element of relaxation which can also be elicited by means of specific breathing techniques. Expiration, generally, is the relaxation phase of respiration. Consequently, encouraging deeper inspiration phases and a free expiration phase can help the body to relax, resulting in the muscle group being treated relaxing further.

Performing the MET stretch technique

1 Post-isometric relaxation (PIR)

- Contraction of the stretched muscle is performed with moderate force.
- Client resists the force against the position if the joint is positioned in flexion. Client must attempt to extend the joint.
- Hold this position for approximately ten seconds.
- Relax the muscle for two seconds before carrying out a further stretch in a slow and progressive manner. This phase should elicit a new barrier position.
- Hold this position for five to ten seconds.

2 Reciprocal inhibition (RI)

- Contraction of the opposing muscle to the stretched muscle.
- If the joint is flexed, to stretch the muscle your client needs to maintain this position against a resistant force.
- Once your client releases the contraction then the muscle is stretched to a new barrier position.
- The technique should be carried out until no further progress can be made. At the final stage of this technique, the new position needs to be held for twenty seconds.

Strengthening techniques

The muscles of the body work very hard to maintain their strength. Sometimes this process is hindered due to injury, illness, damage to other systems, or lack of use. In these cases, the body tries to protect these areas by changing movement patterns and making other muscle groups work harder. This is not always a good thing as it prevents the weaker muscle groups from repairing themselves and recovering or improving.

Muscle fibres need time to adapt to changes in the internal environment, but less time is needed for the nerve supply to the muscle tissue that has become weak to adapt. Therefore increased stimulation of the nerve supply to the weaker muscles can help increase muscular strength. The nerve supply can be stimulated through contraction of the muscle tissue. As the muscle tissue becomes stronger, the use of this specific muscle increases.

! MET FACT

It is vital that communication between you and your client continues throughout the treatment. Your client can give you essential information about the sensation (proprioceptive sense) of the stretches being carried out.

- After your client has contracted the stretched muscle the sensation of the mild stretch should disappear.
- An increase in the sensation of the stretch is the result of the muscle contracting too quickly, the contraction being too strong, or the position that the limb is being held at over-stretching the muscle.

! MET FACT

This technique should not be used on a muscle that has recently experienced an acute injury, as this may result in further damage to the muscle tissue.

! MET FACT

This RI technique should not be used if the opposing muscle will go through contraction in a shortened position. This can result in the antagonistic muscle experiencing muscle spasms (cramps).

Performing the MET strength technique

☐ The weak muscle needs to be stretched to a point before the barrier.

☐ As you apply a controlled force, your client pushes or pulls against the force.

☐ When this technique is used initially, your client should perform concentric contractions (shortening of the agonistic muscle). As strength increases, eccentric contractions (lengthening of the muscle) can be used.

☐ Perform this technique slowly.

Break-down techniques

These techniques are used to help with the smooth action of muscle fibres during contraction and relaxation. Through injury, muscle fibres can become tough and bond together, which hinders the contraction and relaxation of the muscle tissue. This technique attempts to apply a force that will separate these fibres.

To remove adhesive and fibrous tissue, a combination of contraction and stretch techniques is used.

☐ Your client contracts the muscle tissue while the limb is in a shortened position.

☐ You apply a greater force against the force of your client and stretch the muscle. The limb is also moved out and away.

☐ When your client contracts a muscle during extension, you force the joint into flexion.

☐ The force is applied between the fibres with the aim of separating the fibres.

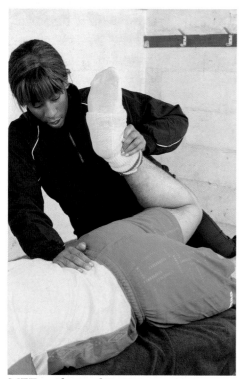

MET on the quadriceps

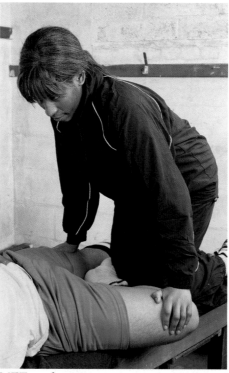

MET on the groin

> **! MET FACT**
>
> This technique can cause considerable damage: if too much force is applied or if the technique is incorrect, torn muscle fibres will result.

> **▶ KNOWLEDGE CHECK**
>
> 1 Describe palpation.
>
> 2 When is palpation used in sports massage?
>
> 3 What use do vibrations have in sports massage?
>
> 4 Name the two types of vibrations.
>
> 5 What are the uses of frictions in sports massage?
>
> 6 What are the differences between circular and transverse frictions?
>
> 7 Describe the steps involved in strain counter strain.
>
> 8 What is neuromuscular technique used for?
>
> 9 What are the benefits of using neuromuscular technique?
>
> 10 Describe one muscle energy technique.

Mechanical
massage

Mechanical massagers are professional instruments that have been designed to simulate the many different techniques of a manual massage. Mechanical massagers work by deeply manipulating muscle tissue and can be used as part of a manual sports massage treatment. There are many different types of mechanical massagers on the market today and there are even some that 'claim' to remove all muscular aches and pains. Mechanical massagers come in all shapes and sizes; some provide heat via an infrared bulb, and others have interchangeable heads.

Mechanical massagers can be bought from many different outlets including catalogues and chemists. Those purchased from these outlets are usually small and for personal use only, and are not suitable for prolonged professional treatments.

Mechanical massagers fall into two categories: gyrators and percussion vibrators.

Gyrators

Floor-standing gyrators

There are two types of gyratory massagers: floor-standing and hand-held. The most common floor-standing massager is the G5.

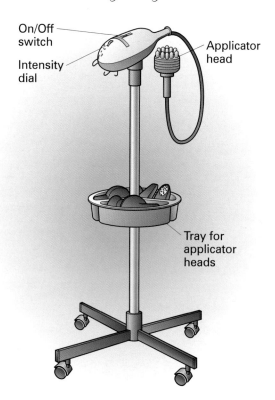

Figure 10.1 The G5

The G5 is a powerful gyratory vibrator, which can be used in combination with a manual sports massage to provide deep tissue manipulation. The G5, with its many different applicator heads, works on two planes: vertical and horizontal.

The movement created by the vertical plane is up and down, whereas the movement created by the horizontal plane is circular and will produce similar effects to a manual massage. By changing applicator heads it can also be used to simulate the effects of effleurage, petrissage and tapotement.

Massage techniques simulated by the G5 applicator heads

The table below illustrates the applicator heads used with the G5 and the massage techniques they simulate.

Name of applicator head	Diagram of applicator head	Massage techniques simulated	Where to use on the body
Contoured sponge		Superficial/deep effleurage; deep stroking	Legs, thighs
Round sponge		Superficial/deep effleurage; deep stroking	Legs, thighs, back, buttocks, shoulders
M		Deep stroking	A contoured applicator to be used in areas where it fits comfortably
Egg cup		Petrissage	Erector spinae (spine sits in between the two rows of balls)
Spike head (short prongs)		Tapotement	Thighs, calf, back, shoulders, buttocks, triceps, biceps
Long prickly prongs		Deep kneading	Muscular areas
Dome		Deep petrissage (will give a superficial massage when intensity is decreased)	Thighs, calf, back, shoulders, buttocks, (triceps, biceps, if muscular)
Lighthouse		Use of thumb	Smaller muscle groups; trigger points
Multi-ball (five or six balls)		Petrissage; deep manipulations	Very muscular areas
Cone		Use of thumb	Trigger points

Advantages and disadvantages of using the G5

There are many advantages and disadvantages of using the G5 in sports massage; they are listed in the table below.

Advantages	Disadvantages
It can simulate some aspects of a manual massage	Treatment may feel very impersonal as the therapist's hands are not in contact with the client
It can provide a deep and stimulating massage	Clients may not feel comfortable with the vibrations produced
Applicator heads can be quickly changed to achieve the desired effect	The noise can be off-putting to the client
The therapist can control the pressure and depth of the vibrations; G5s usually have a dial to control the depth of the vibrations	It can be expensive to purchase
The therapist can treat many clients without becoming unduly tired	It should not be used on bony areas of the body
It can save the therapist time: a full body massage using a G5 may only take twenty minutes compared to 45–60 minutes for a manual massage	It should not be used on clients who have a very slim and bony structure
It can be used in combination with a manual massage	
It can be profitable for the therapist, since more clients can be treated in a day	

Hand-held gyrators

The most common hand-held gyrator is the Heavy Duty Masseter, which, like the G5, produces vibrations; however, because of its size it can be more tiring to use. It, too, has applicator heads that can be used to simulate the effects of massage but they are not as varied as the G5.

The hand-held Heavy Duty Masseter usually has three or four heads, which simulate effleurage, petrissage and tapotement.

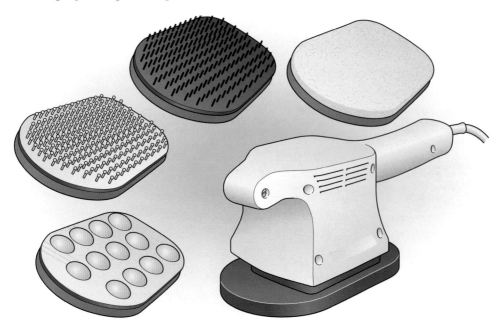

***Figure** 10.2 Hand-held Heavy Duty Masseter with heads*

! GYRATORY FACT

The advantages and disadvantages of using the Heavy Duty Masseter are the same as those listed for the G5 with the addition of the following.

Advantages	Disadvantages
It usually has two settings, which will provide a superficial or deep penetration	The therapist may become tired using the Masseter because of its weight
	Due to its size, use is limited to the large muscular areas of the body

Effects of gyratory massage

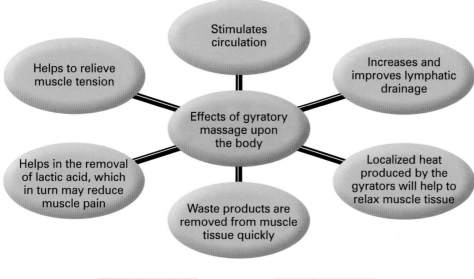

Figure 10.3 *Beneficial effects of gyratory massage*

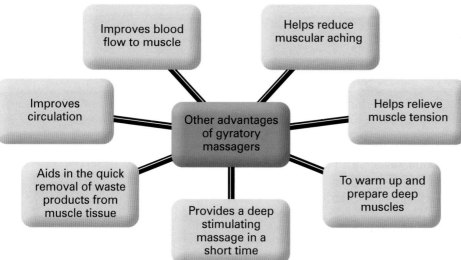

Figure 10.4 *Other advantages of gyratory massagers*

Percussion vibrators

A percussion vibrator is an electrical hand-held device that is used to massage the small muscular areas of the body. A percussion vibrator produces an up-and-down, tapping motion on the skin, which is similar to the percussion or tapotement techniques of a manual massage. Like the G5 and the Heavy Duty Masseter, it has different applicator heads (but not as many as the G5). There is usually a dial on the handle which allows you to increase and decrease the intensity of the vibrations.

Because of its size and the size of the applicator heads, a percussion vibrator can be used effectively on the small muscular areas of the body such as the sternocleidomastoid muscles in the neck, and the deltoids, around the shoulders.

Treatment time varies according to your client's needs; an initial treatment should last between five and ten minutes. Once you have used a percussion vibrator as a form of treatment, you will be able to see how the tissue responds to it and then decide on a course of treatment, increasing the time to no more than 25 minutes.

The tapping effect of the vibrator on the tissue results in the skin becoming red due to the increased blood flow to the area. This is known as erythema.

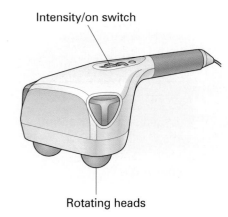

Intensity/on switch

Rotating heads

Figure 10.5
A *percussion vibrator*

Advantages and disadvantages of using a percussion vibrator in sports massage

The advantages and disadvantages of using a percussion vibrator in sports massage are as follows.

Advantages	Disadvantages
It simulates the effects of tapotement	It is less effective than the G5
It can be used on small muscle groups	
It has different applicator heads	It does not have a wide range of applicator heads

Percussion vibrators have been used both in beauty therapy treatments and sports massage for years; there are now many variations on the market today, some of which are more effective than others.

The Audio Sonic

The Audio Sonic is also known as the Audio Sound and is another instrument that is frequently used in sports massage. This appliance produces sound wave vibrations, which can provide a deep muscular penetration of two to three inches.

The Audio Sonic vibrator works by producing sound waves, which are able to run along the length of the muscle tissue. Inside the Audio Sonic is a magnet and situated between the poles of the magnet is a coil which vibrates while moving backwards and forwards as alternating current passes through it. When the Audio Sonic is used on areas of muscle tissue, a deep penetrative vibration is produced.

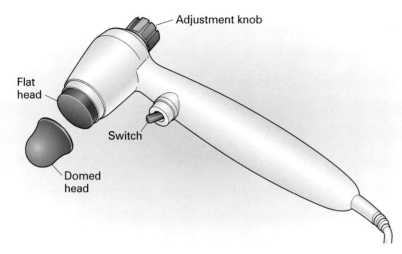

Figure 10.6 Audio Sonic vibrator

Beneficial effects of the Audio Sonic

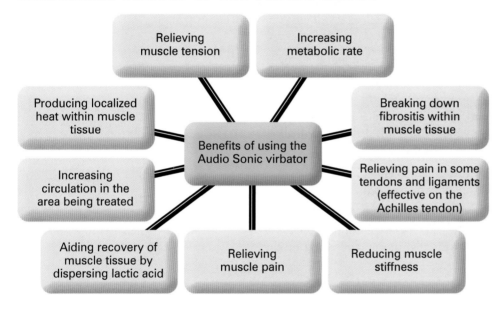

Figure 10.7 Benefits of using the Audio Sonic vibrator

As with percussion vibrators, the Audio Sonic has a dial that allows you to increase or decrease the depth of the vibrations into the muscle tissue. Because of its size and its penetrative ability, the Audio Sonic can be used on small muscular groups as well as being effective in regions of trauma, soreness or tension in the large muscular groups of the body.

How long you will use the Audio Sonic in one treatment session will depend upon the condition of the muscle tissue that is to be treated. Due to the type of vibrations that are produced, the Audio Sonic can be used for up to 25 minutes per session.

Preparing to use the Audio Sonic

As with gyratory and percussion vibrators, talc is required for a smooth application. Run the Audio Sonic over a small area using small circular movements. After treatment, always wash the heads in an anti-bacterial solution.

Contraindications to Audio Sonic massage

The contraindications are the same as those given for gyratory massage.

> **! AUDIO SONIC FACT**
>
> Always finish off with a manual massage. During this manual phase, assess with your hand, using effleurage or stroking, how effective the Audio Sonic treatment has been. In some cases, you may not notice a difference straight away.

Preparing your client for mechanical massage

As always, before performing any type of massage, you should take a full client history. Once you have ascertained that your client has no contraindications to mechanical treatment, explain the treatment to your client so that he or she is not unduly surprised when you switch on the massager.

Preparation for mechanical massage

1 Ensure that your client is positioned safely and comfortably on the couch and that the body areas not being treated are covered with towels.

2 Apply talc to the surface of the skin. Talcum powder allows the applicator heads to run smoothly over the surface of the skin. Never use oil, as it will clog up the applicator heads, especially the sponge heads.

3 Start by using an effleurage pad. Switch the machine on low and hold the pad in your hand; this is to ensure that the pad is fitted correctly and is secure.

4 Transfer the pad quickly and smoothly from your hand to your client's leg, and perform an effleurage, using an upward, sweeping movement, following the contours of the leg. Perform four to six strokes using this pad. This will allow your client to get used to the vibrations and the specific treatment.

5 Use a petrissage pad next to perform a kneading movement. When changing applicator heads, turn away from your client and change them quickly and efficiently.

6 Always work towards the heart and use this pad in a circular motion; always apply pressure on the upward stroke of the circular movement. Never tilt the pad; always keep it parallel to the skin.

7 Change to a pad that produces similar effects to tapotement, again working in a circular motion and with the venous return.

8 Always finish off the treatment using the effleurage pad.

9 Remove any remaining talc from the surface of the skin.

10 Apply oil or cream and finish off with a manual massage. This will allow you to feel how effective the mechanical massager has been and to determine whether more treatment is required. It will also allow your client to feel your own personal touch.

Introducing mechanical massage

It may be a good idea to introduce your client to the vibrations of a mechanical massager – once you have explained the intended treatment – by letting him or her feel them before beginning the full treatment. Discuss the sensations he or she will feel and then slowly move the massager on a low setting over the body area being treated.

Length of time to use each pad

Once you have assessed your client by means of communication, observation and palpation, you will then have to decide how long to use each pad for. Use it for three to four minutes in the first instance. The length of time will depend on the condition of the muscle and the reason why your client needs treatment.

> **! GYRATORY FACT**
>
> Remember, you do not have to use all of the pads. You may just choose the ones that you feel may be the most effective. Always combine mechanical massage treatment with a manual massage.

Care of the interchangeable heads

After each use, always wash the heads in hot water and an anti-bacterial solution in order to prevent any cross-infection occurring. Allow the heads to dry naturally.

CONTRAINDICATION TO MECHANICAL MASSAGE

Do not use a mechanical massager if your client:

☐ has an infectious skin disorder, such as impetigo

☐ has inflamed areas of skin or muscle tissue

☐ has varicose veins

☐ has paralysed muscles

☐ is pregnant or menstruating (do not use on the stomach)

☐ has a very bony frame

☐ has bruises

☐ has very hairy skin

☐ has areas of broken skin.

▶ KNOWLEDGE CHECK

1 Name the different types of mechanical massagers.

2 What is a gyrator?

3 The G5 has many different applicator heads. Name five and identify the manual massage technique that each simulates.

4 Give five advantages of using the G5 in sports massage.

5 Describe the Heavy Duty Masseter.

6 What effects do gyrators have upon the body?

7 What are the contraindications to mechanical massage?

8 What are the advantages and disadvantages of using the percussion vibrator in sports massage?

9 How does the Audio Sonic work and what are its uses in sports massage?

10 What are the contraindications to Audio Sonic massage?

Injuries

Classification of injuries

Participation in regular physical exercise, maintaining all aspects of fitness, and recovery through rest and physical therapy can all help to maintain a well-balanced body. Injuries may, nevertheless, occur during physical activity. It is the responsibility of both coach and athlete to recognize that an injury has occurred and to evaluate the extent of this injury; this is only possible if you have a thorough knowledge of related anatomy and physiology.

The many injuries that occur in sport are caused in a number of different ways. Injuries can be classed as:

☐ accidental injuries

☐ overuse injuries

☐ chronic injuries.

The factors that cause either accidental or overuse injuries may be internal (force from within the body) or external (force from outside the body).

Injuries can be divided into primary and secondary injuries.

Injury	Cause
Primary consequential	Direct result of the sport or action
Secondary non-consequential	Lack of exercise because of injury

Some injuries come under the heading of trauma.

Trauma	Examples of trauma
Macro trauma – acute injury from event	Fractures, dislocations/subluxation, a single sprain, strains, contusions, abrasions, cuts
Micro trauma – overuse, cumulative	Tendonitis, traction, bursitis, stress fractures

Once an acute injury has been identified, it is important to evaluate and determine what to do next. In the first instance, basic first-aid steps should be taken. These are:

☐ assess the situation

☐ determine whether the limb can be moved; if not, make your client as comfortable as possible and then call for an ambulance

☐ if the limb can be moved, the RICE method (rest, ice, compression, elevation) can be followed.

Levels of pain

Levels of pain due to injury can be categorized in the following way.

Ligaments

Degree of pain	Disruption of fibres	Level of laxity
Mild	None	None
Moderate	Some	Some
Severe	Total	Total

Muscles

Degree of pain	Disruption of fibres	Level of laxity
Mild	None	Pain, no weakness; full range of movement
Moderate	Moderate	Pain and weakness; limited range of movement; pain on passive stretching
Severe	Total	Little or no range of movement; severe pain on passive stretching

Injury observation

Injury observation includes the following criteria. Look for any area of:

☐ pain

☐ swelling

☐ restrictions

☐ weakness

☐ noise and creaking (crepitation) in the area.

Next, determine the degree of pain during movement. Determine when the pain is at its worst, for example, during active flexion or stretching of the muscle, or during passive restrictions. Test for an imbalance or limitation during movement.

Having corrected the necessary information through the above process, you should advise or carry out (if qualified) the appropriate treatment. However, as mentioned previously, you must apply basic first-aid treatment in the case of acute injuries.

Methods of collecting client information

Listen	Look	Touch
How did the injury happen?	Signs	Texture
When did the injury occurr?	Symptoms	Heat
	Abnormalities	Range of motion – active and passive
Appearance	Pallor	Laxity
Has the injury happened before?	Size and/or bulk	Power
Immediate treatment required?	Swelling	Stability
Further treatment required?	Active range of motion	Sensation

The RICE method

This is one of the most important elements of injury management. It can reduce the swelling of the injured site and help in the recovery process.

Rest

The client must stop using the injured area as soon as an injury has occurred, avoid weight-bearing activities, use crutches if he or she has a lower body injury, or get help to move to an appropriate location.

Ice

Ice packs can be applied to help stop or reduce internal bleeding of the injured area. Internal bleeding is due to blood vessels such as capillaries being damaged. The cold ice causes these small vessels to contract, resulting in reduced blood flow which prevents blood from collecting around the injured site.

Application of ice

- Iced water in a bucket can be used for small injuries to phalanges, (meta)tarsals and (meta)carpals.
- Ice packs can be used on injuries to large areas of the body. These packs can be made from ice cubes placed in a bag. Place the ice pack in a towel or cloth covering and then place on the skin where the injury has occurred.
- See also Ice massage in the glossary on page xxx.

Compression

Fluid from neighbouring areas can bleed into the injured area delaying recovery of the damaged tissues. Compression helps to reduce the amount of swelling around an injured area.

- Use elasticated bandages for compression or wrap the area with a cloth. The wrapping should be firm and include the ice pack if possible.
- If the area becomes blue and a feeling of pain, numbness or cramps is experienced, then remove the wrapping immediately, as these are signs of a lack of blood in the area, a factor which will also hinder recovery.

Elevation

Elevation is also used to reduce swelling. Elevate the injured part above heart level to help in venous return. Pillows or solid objects can be used to support the area.

If the limb can be moved, the MICER (mobilization, ice, compression, elevation, rest) method can be implemented. The degree of mobility needs to be assessed by moving the limb normally. Never attempt this if a fracture or broken bone is suspected.

! ICE FACT

It is vital to remember not to place ice and ice packs directly onto the skin, as this can cause ice burns.

- The ice pack should remain on the injury for approximately twenty minutes and then be removed.
- Allow the area to regain some heat for fifteen minutes and then reapply the ice pack. This process should be continued for up to three hours after the injury has happened.
- If pain and swelling continue, refer to a medical professional.

Rehabilitation

The aim of rehabilitation after an injury is to aid an individual to return to their state of fitness aspects prior to the injury. The rehabilitation phase of recovery focuses on all aspects of fitness, strength, flexibility and endurance. The rehabilitation of the injured part of the body usually takes place once the inflammation of an injured site has reduced considerably (between 24 and 72 hours after injury).

> **! REHABILITATION FACT**
>
> Rehabilitation of the injured part should also be combined with exercising the rest of the body.

Rehabilitation programmes should not be followed after serious injuries, such as fractures, dislocations or severe sprains, without clearance from doctors or consultants.

Rehabilitation programmes are designed in consultation with your client, with sports therapy or massage techniques, exercise, and prescriptive and non-prescriptive medical agents all being taken into consideration. It is important to note that the sports massage therapist cannot prescribe any medical agent for an injury.

Goals should be set for massage and exercise and your client's progress monitored throughout treatment.

Rehabilitation treatments include:

- saunas, steam baths, spa pools and hydrotherapy baths, ultraviolet and infrared, radiant heat: these are classed as heat treatments
- gyratherapy
- Audio Sonic vibrators
- percussion vibrators
- sports massage.

The healing process

There are three phases to the healing process: acute, repair, and remodelling. There are various factors that will determine how long the injury will take to repair.

The acute phase

This can be classed as the initial phase of treatment to an injury.

Treatment during the acute phase aims to reduce the flow of blood to the injured site. This helps to minimize the amount of swelling around the area. The RICE method is usually used during this stage of healing. Gentle movement should also be encouraged.

The repair phase

The repair phase begins on the third day after the injury has occurred when the swelling of the area has reduced. At this point, essential nutrients, delivered to the site of the injury, begin to repair the damaged tissues. As muscle tissue is unable to replace itself, scar tissue is formed. Scar tissue is not as strong or as flexible as the original muscle tissue, therefore muscle function is reduced. Treatment during this phase attempts to increase the strength and elasticity of the new tissue.

Ice

Ice is used to restrict blood flow to an area. Once this is removed, there is an increase of blood flow to the area as the vessels dilate. The consequent increase of nutrients in the blood during this stage helps to initiate healing.

Massage

Effleurage has been found to be the most appropriate massage technique for this stage, as deeper and more vigorous techniques may cause further damage to the area.

Stretching

Stretching can promote elasticity of the scarred muscle tissue.

Gentle resistance exercises

These types of exercises help to improve the strength of the muscle tissue in the injured area. The use of light weights or isometric exercises, where muscles are encouraged to contract without producing movement, is appropriate at this stage.

The remodelling phase

The remodelling phase is the final phase of rehabilitation. It may be a long-term process during which the scar tissue increases in strength and suppleness during movement. Massage techniques during this phase can be much deeper and firmer. Strength training programmes can be used along with developmental stretches. Stability exercises can help to stimulate damaged nerve endings.

The recovery process should include educating your client in the prevention or reoccurrence of injury. Knowledge of correct warm-up and cool-down procedures should be reinforced, along with information on adequate and appropriate flexibility and strength exercises, and correct techniques.

A–Z of sports injuries

Adductor strain

Sport	Badminton
Causes	Quick changes in direction during running, taking the adductor muscle beyond the point of alignment or range of motion.
Signs and symptoms	Sharp pain in the groin area which may increase as the activity continues. There will also be weakness during flexion of the hip and adduction movements.
Treatment	Immediate ice treatments should be carried out. After the initial pain has disappeared, ice methods should be used during static stretching. Continue with static passive stretching and gentle massage to reduce discomfort.

Ankle sprain

Sport	Basketball
Causes	Stress on either side of the ankle joint, which then forces the ankle from its normal alignment. The ligaments that hold the joint in place are torn or over-stretched.
Signs and symptoms	There is pain in the ankle joint at the time of the injury. There may also be a feeling of popping or tearing in the outer region of the ankle joint.
Other symptoms	Swelling and tenderness in the area. With slight injuries to the ankle joint there is slight loss of function. This loss of function increases the more severe the injury. Bruising usually appears a few hours after the injury has occurred.
Treatment	After the initial treatment of the area, ice massage the injury three to four times a day in 20-minute sessions. After 72 hours, apply heat treatments and elevate the limb whenever possible. Massage the ankle area with gentle movements once the swelling has reduced.

Ankle tenosynovitis

Sport	Skiing
Causes	Strain from an unusual use of the ankle or possible overuse of the soft tissues of the area, or a direct blow to the ankle area.
Signs and symptoms	Pain felt during movement and limited movement of the area. Heat and redness may be experienced over the area of the damaged tendon.

Treatment	Heat treatment after the initial care. Exercises will help to strengthen the area only after supportive strapping is no longer required. Use ice massage techniques for ten minutes before and after exercise.

Arm exostosis (blocker's exostosis)

Sport	Rugby
Causes	Repeated injury to the upper arm (humerus). Injuries can include sprains and strains or chronic irritation of an already damaged bone.
Signs and symptoms	Pain and tenderness at the site of the overgrowth of the bone. Pain during pressure exerted on the upper arm. Possible change of the line of the humerus ranging from a slight lump to a large spur.
Treatment	Immediate use of RICE. Support the arm to reduce the weight loading of the arm. Heat treatments such as ultrasound or aquatherapy can be employed. Protective clothing should be worn if participation continues.

Back sprain of the lumbo-sacro region

Sport	Weight-lifting
Causes	Direct blow or stress on the ligaments of the lumbo-sacro region. The force of the action of lifting weights forces the sacroiliac joints from their normal alignment.
Signs and symptoms	Pain at time of injury with a feeling that the muscle has been torn. There will be tenderness and swelling at the injury site. Bruising is visible soon after the injury has occurred.
Treatment	Use ice packs three to four times per day within 72 hours of the injury. Bandage the area between treatments. After 72 hours, heat treatments can be administered. Gentle massage can also help to reduce swelling and relieve discomfort.

Bicep strain

Sport	Archery
Causes	Prolonged overuse of the bicep muscle and the tendons of the area when drawing back the bow. A sudden or single violent blow to the area can also cause damage.
Signs and symptoms	Pain during flexion and extension of the bicep muscle can be experienced. There may also be visible swelling around the injury. In some cases, crepitation can be heard when the injury is pressed with the fingers.

Treatment	Ice massage the area three to four times per day in 15-minute sessions. Twenty-four hours after the injury, heat treatments can be used, as well as gentle massage over the area if there is no swelling or disfigurement of the bicep muscle.

Bicipital tendonitis

Sport	Canoeing
Causes	Repetitive and rapid overhead movements when taking the paddle through the rotation of the stroke. Excessive flexion and supination of the elbow and arm.
Signs and symptoms	Irritation of the bicep tendon. Pain and tenderness when the shoulder internally and externally rotates. Pain during passive stretching when the shoulder and elbow are extended and the forearm is pronated.
Treatment	Restrict rotational movements. Take the weight by using a sling when at resting state. Heat and electrical therapy can be used. Ice therapy can be used before and after activity; flexibility and strength exercises should also be carried out.

Bursitis

Sport	Badminton
Causes	Injury often occurs when an individual falls with a bent knee. Possible causes are arthritis and gout or infections in the knee bursa.
Signs and symptoms	Tenderness when moving the area and in some cases pain during movement. Swelling occurs around the area and the affected bursa often shows signs of redness. There is also limited movement in the problem area.
Treatment	Ice massage methods can be used. Load-bearing movements should not be carried out. After 72 hours, heat treatments may be used if preferred. Elevate the knee whenever possible. Gentle massage can help reduce swelling.

Carpal tunnel syndrome

Sport	Judo
Causes	Repetitive overuse of the wrist and finger flexors. There is a thickening of the synovial covering of the carpal tendons. Inflammation due to constant gripping or squeezing.
Signs and symptoms	Morning stiffness of the wrist. Numbness and tingling may be felt in the thumb, index and middle fingers. A burning sensation may also be experienced. Grip strength decreases and the hand is unable to form a fist.

Treatment	Immobilization of the wrist especially during extension. Use ice massage to reduce swelling. Possible surgery to release any nerves that may be trapped.

Dead-leg or 'Charley Horse'

Sport	Soccer
Causes	Single direct force during contact with a blunt object, a person or equipment.
Signs and symptoms	Swelling appears over the trauma, and superficial bruising tracking down towards the knee can be seen soon after the injury has occurred. There is tenderness and warmth in the area and limited movement during flexion and extension of the thigh.
Treatment	RICE is the initial treatment. For the first 24 hours, ice treatment can be used, especially during flexion of the knee and hip. A bandage can be used to restrict further damage to the area.

NB No massage should be given, no vigorous stretching or exercise should be used, and heat treatments such as ultrasound should be avoided.

Finger numbness injury: ulnar neuropathy and cyclist palsy

Sport	Cycling
Causes	Inflammation of Guyon's canal places pressure on the ulnar nerve, due to repetitive trauma to the palmar aspect of the hand. It is caused by the cyclist leaning on the handlebars of the bike for an extended period of time.
Signs and symptoms	Feeling of numbness in the little finger. Inability to pick up light objects, particularly with the thumb and index finger. In cyclist palsy, the symptoms may disappear soon after the race or ride.
Treatment	Rest and heat treatments may help to alleviate the symptoms but if these continue beyond six months then further assistance from a medical professional will be required.

Foot ganglion (synovial hernia, synovial cyst)

Sport	Skiing
Causes	Mild or chronic sprains of the foot joints, which weaken the joint capsules. A problem with the fibrous sheath of the joint or tendon can lead to the synovium (thin membrane of the tendon) coming through. The synovium may become irritated so that the area fills with fluid.

Signs and symptoms	A hard lump appears over a tendon or joint in the foot. Overuse of the foot may result in pain and tenderness in the area if pressure is exerted on it.
Treatment	In severe cases, surgery may be necessary; after the wounds have healed, ice massage or heat treatments can be used.

Game-keeper's thumb

Sport	Cricket
Causes	The joint of the thumb is abducted forcefully away from the hand.
Signs and symptoms	This injury is very painful and the area very swollen. Instability of the thumb occurs during movements of flexion and extension.
Treatment	Immediate treatment with ice and immobilization techniques. For mild cases, mobilization and ultrasound can be used.

Golfer's elbow (medial epicondylitis)

Sport	Golf
Causes	Repeated tensions during the follow-through of a swing causes tears in the wrist flexors and the pronator muscle group. The injury also occurs in javelin throwing after the release of the javelin. Overhead actions aggravate the elbow region.
Signs and symptoms	Pain at the medial aspect of the ulnar collateral ligaments. Possible popping and tearing sound in severe injuries. A sharp pain is experienced during overhead movements. If the ulnar nerve is affected by the injury, tingling and numbness of the area may be felt.
Treatment	Avoid overhead movements for up to twelve weeks. The use of ice massage and ultrasound can be beneficial. Frictions massage over the flexor tendon can help reduce the viscosity of the tendon.

Hamstring strain

Sport	Hockey
Causes	Rapid contraction of the muscle group during a ballistic movement or when the muscle is overstretched in a violent manner.
Other causes include	Poor flexibility of the muscle; imbalance of the muscle group; poor posture.
Signs and symptoms	Pain when the hip is in flexion and the knee is extended. Muscle spasm may occur and swelling over the injured area.

Treatment	Active stretching needs to be carried out and strengthening of both the quadriceps and the hamstrings is essential. Ice massage can be used at first and then heat treatments 24 hours after the initial injury. Reduce the discomfort by using gentle massage frequently.

Hand sprain

Sport	Gymnastics
Causes	Falling or pressing on an outstretched hand when performing a skill; the hand joints are forced from their normal alignment and this damages the ligaments.
Signs and symptoms	Pain in the joints of the hand at the time of the injury. There may also be a feeling of popping or tearing in the region. Swelling and tenderness over the area and a slight loss of function. Bruising usually appears a few hours after the injury has occurred.
Treatment	If a cast is not required, ice massage techniques can be applied. After 72 hours, heat treatment can replace the ice massage. Frequent gentle massage can help to reduce the swelling.

Hand strain

Sport	Riding
Causes	Prolonged overuse of the muscle tendons in the forearm, wrist or hand. Strains can also be caused by a violent force being applied to the region.
Signs and symptoms	Cramp, fatigue, muscle spasm and pain in the affected hand muscles can be experienced, along with pain during movement and stretching of the hand. Swelling and tenderness may also be experienced.
Treatment	Ice massage, heat treatments and gentle massage can all be used. Healing of soft tissues sometimes takes as long as skeletal fractures: mild strains take between two and ten days, whereas severe strains can take up to ten weeks to repair.

Impingement syndrome

Sport	Swimming
Causes	Overuse of repetitive overhead movements.
Signs and symptoms	Pain during overhead movements when the shoulder rotates externally and internally. Snapping or clicking during the shoulder movements and weakness of the shoulder and the bicep.

Treatment	Restricting range of movement to below 90 degrees of abduction. Ultrasound, ice therapy and heat treatments can also be beneficial. Progressive resistant exercises can help to strengthen the injured area.

Knee sprain

Sport	Badminton
Causes	The knee may move out of its normal position, thereby placing stress on the ligaments around the knee area.
Signs and symptoms	Severe pain at the time of the injury occurring, with a popping feeling inside the knee joint.
Other symptoms	Tenderness and swelling around the injured area. Some bruising may appear.
Treatment	After initial immobilization of the knee joint, ice packs can reduce swelling and inflammation in the area. After 72 hours, heat treatments and gentle massage can be applied at frequent intervals to help reduce the swelling.

Lower leg (calf) (tennis leg) strain

Sport	Soccer
Causes	Prolonged use of the muscle tendons of the calf or a single force applied to the area.
Signs and symptoms	Pain when moving the foot or ankle joint during stretching.
Other symptoms	Muscle spasm at the injury site; swelling may appear. Crepitation (crackling) may be heard when the area is pressed.
Treatment	Support the lower leg with an elastic tube. Some cases require the leg to be placed in a splint or cast. The toes need to be free so that exercises can be carried out. Ice massage can be used after basic first-aid treatment. Heat treatments can be used if preferred. Massage gently for comfort and elevate the leg whenever possible.

Lumbar back strain

Sport	Rowing
Causes	Lumbar muscles counteract the movements for bending forward during performing a technique. The entire trunk is flexed forward, which places a strain on the lumbar region.
Signs and symptoms	Pain is experienced in the specific area of injury. This pain continues as the activity continues.
Treatment	Rest and heat treatments. Gentle massage to stretch the muscle tissue and to reduce tension and discomfort.

Neck sprain

Sport	Gymnastics
Causes	Violent overstretching of the neck ligaments that forces the joints out of their normal location. If the injury involves more than a single ligament, then more disability will occur.
Signs and symptoms	Severe pain at the time of the injury and a sound of tearing in the neck region. Soreness of the neck and possible muscle spasm. The neck will be tender to touch and swelling will be visible, with bruising around the area.
Treatment	RICE for immediate treatment. The doctor may suggest a brace to support the neck during the healing process. Ice massage can be used for up to 72 hours. After this, heat treatments and gentle massage can be used. Do **not** massage over the vertebrae.

Neck strain

Sport	Rugby
Causes	Overuse of the muscle tendons in the neck or a single force applied to the area. Overuse during a scrum of the neck muscle that attaches to the shoulder region. A single force may come from contact in a scrum or a tackle.
Signs and symptoms	Pain during movement or stretching of the neck. Swelling occurs around the neck region and strength is reduced.
Treatment	Simply rest, but RICE for immediate treatment. Ice massage techniques can be used for up to 24 hours. Heat treatments can be used after this time with gentle massage to increase comfort and decrease swelling. Do **not** massage over the vertebrae.

Olecranon bursitis

Sport	Darts, shooting
Causes	Falling on a flexed elbow or from repeated pressure and friction when constantly leaning on the elbow.
Signs and symptoms	Inflammation indicated by heat, redness and swelling.
Treatment	Ice treatments for the initial 24 hours after the injury, followed by heat treatments.

Pectoralis major strain

Sport	Weight-lifting
Causes	Overuse of muscle tendons of the sternum and the ribs, especially during chest press activities.

Signs and symptoms	Pain when moving and pushing the arm and stretching the chest. Muscle spasms occur and swelling around the injured site will appear. There will also be a loss of strength when lifting weights.
Treatment	Ice massage therapy can be used and frequent gentle chest massage.

Pelvis strain (hip–trunk)

Sport	Hockey
Causes	Overuse of the muscle group around the iliac crest or a violent force applied to the muscle tendons in the upper region of the pelvic girdle.
Signs and symptoms	Pain can be felt during moving or stretching the trunk and hip. There may also be muscle spasm at the injury site and swelling may appear. Crepitation (crackling) may be heard when the area is pressed.
Treatment	After basic first-aid, ice massage can be used, followed after 24 hours, by heat treatments. Use gentle massage around the area to help reduce swelling.

Quadriceps strain

Sport	Weight-lifting
Causes	Overuse of the quadriceps or the muscle tendons of the muscle group or a single violent force applied to the area. Overuse of the muscle tendons from the repetitive action of squatting or using the legs to push the weights above the head. A single force from the quick action of lifting heavy weights above the head.
Signs and symptoms	Pain during flexion of the upper leg. Pain and swelling of the quadriceps and loss of strength. There may also be inflammation of the tendon sheath of the quadriceps.
Treatment	Ice massage techniques for up to 24 hours, or heat treatments if more comfortable. Gentle massage can also be used to reduce swelling and increase comfort. Rehabilitation exercises can be used after support is no longer required.

Runner's knee (chondromalacia patellae)

Sport	Basketball
Causes	Muscle imbalance or compression at the knee joint. This pulls the kneecap away and sideways from the natural alignment.

Signs and symptoms	Soreness or aching around the kneecap or under the kneecap. These feelings become worse if activities such as walking, running or jumping continue. Sometimes the knee may give way or develop water on the knee.
Treatment	Use ice packs and ice treatments. These can then be substituted with heat treatments. Strengthening of the hamstrings and the quadriceps muscle group may also be necessary.

Shoulder sprain (gleno-humeral)

Sport	Boxing
Causes	Stress when taking the arm back and upward, moving the shoulder out of alignment. This forces the ligaments and bones to move out of the range or line of movement.
Signs and symptoms	Pain is experienced at the time of injury. There will be a swelling over the area and a loss of strength. A popping or tearing sound may also be heard. Bruising appears soon after the injury has occurred.
Treatment	Ice massage for up to 72 hours, followed by heat treatments. If the injury is not too severe, then continued participation of activity is permissible. Ice massage prior to activity. Gentle massage of shoulder muscle groups helps to reduce the swelling and discomfort.

Shoulder strain

Sport	Rugby
Causes	Overuse of the muscle tendons in the shoulder region during a scrum or any contact move, or a single force to the area.
Signs and symptoms	Pain during movement or stretching of the shoulder area. In some cases, muscle spasm in the shoulder. Swelling of the area and a loss of strength.
Treatment	Ice massage for up to 72 hours, followed by heat treatment. If the injury is not too severe, then continued participation of activity is permissable. Ice massage prior to activity. Frequent gentle massage of the area can also help to reduce swelling and discomfort.

Skater's heel (pump bump)

Sport	Skating
Causes	Excessive pressure around the heel area as a result of the Achilles tendon during plantarflexion pushing off from the ground.

Signs and symptoms	Pain when lifting the heel or during plantarflexion when pushing off from the ground. This movement irritates and inflames the area.
Treatment	Ice massage of the Achilles tendon and the bursa region. Gentle massage treatment to reduce discomfort. Stretching exercises of the Achilles tendon.

Tennis elbow or elbow tendonitis (epicondylitis)

Sport	Tennis
Causes	Partial tears of the tendons attached to the epicondyle. Sudden or chronic stress to the tissues attached to the muscles of the lower arm and the elbow area. Possible reasons are snapping of the wrist when the racquet makes contact with the ball, incorrect grip of the racquet, incorrect technique when hitting the ball, or inappropriate equipment.
Signs and symptoms	Pain or tenderness in the epicondyle, which worsens during rotation of the arm or when attempting to grip an object.
Treatment	After basic first-aid treatment, heat treatments help to relieve the pain. After the pain has disappeared, arm stretches should be performed while wearing a splint over the elbow area.

Tricep strain

Sport	Baseball
Causes	Overuse of the muscles and tendons of the area, from constant extension when throwing the ball, for instance. However, a single force to the area can also cause damage to the soft tissue of the arm and elbow.
Signs and symptoms	Pain is experienced when the elbow is moved or during forceful extension of the forearm at the elbow joint.
Other symptoms	Muscle spasm; swelling around the injured area.
Treatment	Sufficient rest is required to repair the soft tissues. Continue with ice massage techniques three or four times per day and then, after the first 24 hours, apply heat treatments to the area. Gentle massage can be applied once the swelling has disappeared.

Wrist ganglion (synovial hernia, synovial cyst)

Sport	Squash
Causes	Mild or chronic sprains of the wrist joints, which weaken the joint capsules. A problem with the fibrous sheath of the joint or tendon can lead to the synovium (thin membrane of the tendon) breaking through. The synovium may become irritated resulting in the area filling with fluid.
Signs and symptoms	A hard lump appears over a tendon or joint in the wrist. Overuse of the wrist may result in pain and tenderness in the area if pressure is exerted on it.
Treatment	In severe cases, surgery may be necessary; after the wounds have healed, ice massage or heat treatments can be used.

Wrist sprain

Sport	Gymnastics
Causes	Falling or pressing on an outstretched arm when the wrist is hyperflexed. This may occur when force is applied during vaulting or floor exercises.
Signs and symptoms	Pain during the activity and when performing passive extension of the wrist.
Treatment	Decrease the intensity of the training and strap the area. Strength exercises for the forearm can be performed once the pain has subsided.

Many of the following injuries fall into the category of track and field athletics.

Abdominal wall strain

Sport	High jump, triple jump
Causes	Overuse of the muscle tendons during the stretching phases of these activities.
Signs and symptoms	Pain is experienced when moving and stretching the abdominal wall. Muscle spasm occurs when twisting or during hard breathing. Swelling appears over the wall and there is a loss of strength.
Treatment	After 24 hours, use heat treatments instead of ice massage if preferred. Massage gently and often to decrease the swelling.

Achilles tendonitis

Sport	Sprinting
Causes	Repetitive over-extension and overload of the Achilles tendon.
Other causes include	Tight heel cords; a change in footwear or surface when training; increase in distance when running; increase in intensity, that is, speed or steepness of the runs.
Signs and symptoms	Pain occurs before and after activity. This pain will increase during passive stretching exercises of the tendon in dorsiflexion and during plantarflexion when resistance is present.
Treatment	Ice massage of the area and restriction of sports participation for approximately three weeks. Include active stretches of the Achilles tendon during treatment sessions and before and after training. In some cases, heel lift may need to be used in shoes.

Anterior compartment syndrome

Sport	Long-distance running
Causes	Fractures, strains and overuse can cause anterior compartment syndrome.
Signs and symptoms	Lower leg pain during activity, which does not decrease during rest intervals.
Other symptoms include	Increased pain and swelling of the area; muscle bulk increases and the skin becomes tight; loss of sensation between the big toe and the second toe.
Treatment	Ice massage and rest can help to reduce the pain and swelling in the area. If the foot becomes numb, then surgery may be needed. Avoid elevating the leg as this hinders the arterial blood supply to the area.

Back sprain of the lumbo-dorsal region

Sport	Hammer throwing
Causes	Stress on the ligaments of the lumbo-dorsal region, forcing the ligaments out of their normal alignment. A sprain occurs when the weight is excessive or when the athlete is off-balance during the execution of the throw.
Signs and symptoms	Severe pain at time of injury and a possible sound of popping or tearing of the muscle in the lumbo-dorsal region. Tenderness and swelling at the injury site.
Treatment	Use ice packs three to four times per day within 72 hours of the injury occurring. After 72 hours, heat treatments can be administered. Gentle massage can also help to reduce swelling and relieve discomfort.

Jumper's knee – patella tendonitis

Causes	Repetitive knee extensions
Signs and symptoms	Pain occurs after participation in the activity. However, as the injury progresses, pain is experienced at the beginning of the activity; this pain wears off during participation of the activity but is experienced again afterwards. Pain may be felt when walking up and down stairs or after sitting for a period of time.
Treatment	Avoid painful exercises. Use heat treatments such as ultrasound and aquatherapy. Strengthen the quadriceps and hamstrings through eccentric contractions and include stretches of these muscle groups.

Lower leg stress fractures

Sport	Long-distance running
Causes	Overuse of the lower leg, especially of the tibia and fibula. Participation in high-intensity work for a long period of time, often without sufficient recovery time. Changes in the environment, intensity, the footwear of the athlete, and the muscular strength of the lower leg.
Signs and symptoms	Pain in the lower leg is specific to the area of the stress fractures. Warmth and tenderness of the area and swelling over the area.
Categories of pain	**1** Pain is experienced after the activity has finished. **2** Pain is experienced during the activity but may continue afterwards. **3** Pain is not relieved and can be described as chronic.
Treatment	Rest is essential. If pain category 1 is experienced, then decrease the intensity and frequency of training or participation in the activity. If categories 2 and 3 are experienced, training and participation in the activity should be avoided altogether until pain can no longer be felt at the end of each day. Return to former levels of training and participation in the activity should be gradual. Ice massage can be used to help relieve pain, but further massage should not be used as this could increase the pain.

Pelvic strain

Sport	Hurdles
Causes	Overuse of the muscle tendons of the adductors, hamstrings, abdominals and the lower back, for example, during flexion of the hip and the knee in an extended position (as in the leading leg over the hurdles). Strains occur at the weakest part of this region.
Signs and symptoms	Pain is experienced when moving or stretching the leg. Muscle spasms occur at the attachment to the pelvis. There is swelling in the lower pelvic area (ischium).
Treatment	Ice massage of the attachments of the muscle tendons to the ischium. Gentle massage to reduce discomfort and swelling.

Glossary of terms

Acute injury
A single force is directed upon a structure, which produces an injury.

Chronic injury
Repeated force or loading over a period of time, which results in an injury.

Compression
A force is directed along the length of a bone or soft tissue.

Crepitation
A crackling sound produced when the ends of bone meet and move against each other.

Cryotherapy
Therapy using cold application methods to reduce swelling and pain. See also **ice massage**.

Friction massage
Massage performed at an angle to a tissue with the aim of loosening the scar tissue and reducing muscle spasm in the specific area.

Hematoma
A mass of blood and lymph that accumulates within an area of muscle tissue.

Hypermobility
Range of motion of a joint that is greater than average.

Hypomobility
Range of motion of a joint that is smaller than average.

Ice massage
Massage technique using iced water or ice cubes. Either the lid is placed on a foam cup of iced water and this is used to perform massage over the area in circular movements; alternatively, a foam cup is filled with ice cubes until they protrude and this is used to perform the massage. This is usually carried out three or four times per day for approximately fifteen minutes for the initial 24–72 hours after the injury has taken place.

Laceration
A wound that opens the skin and goes through to the subcutaneous layer of the skin, muscles, associated nerves and blood vessels.

Referred pain

Pain that is experienced in an area of the body other than at the original site of the injury.

RICE

Rest, ice, compression, elevation.

Spasm

Temporary muscle contractions.

Sprain

Injury to a soft tissue or ligament i.e. injury to a soft tissue or ligament.

Strain

Injury to a muscle or its tendon. The degree of pain and swelling is due to muscle fibres either being torn or a complete rupture occuring.

Synovitis

Inflammation of the synovial membrane, which surrounds a synovial joint.

Tendonitis

Inflammation of the muscle tendon.

Tenosynovitis

Inflammation of the muscle tendon sheath.

Tension

A force that pulls with the intent to stretch a soft tissue.

Thermotherapy

Therapy using the application of heat.

Torque or bending injury

An injury sustained when force is applied to a structure from opposing directions, which causes it to bend and, in severe cases, fracture.

Ultrasound

Therapy that uses high frequency sound waves. This method should be used only in the second phase of the treatment on injuries, not in the primary phase of treatment.

Index

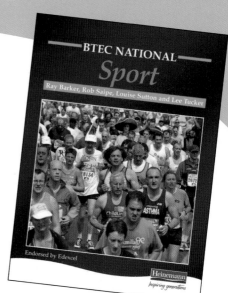
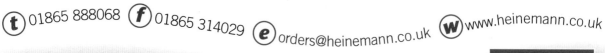
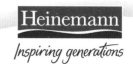